Super Diets Guidebook

An Introduction to the Mediterranean, Keto, Fasting Diets, and More

Kevin Jobson

Table of Contents

Introduction: Super Diets for Your Health

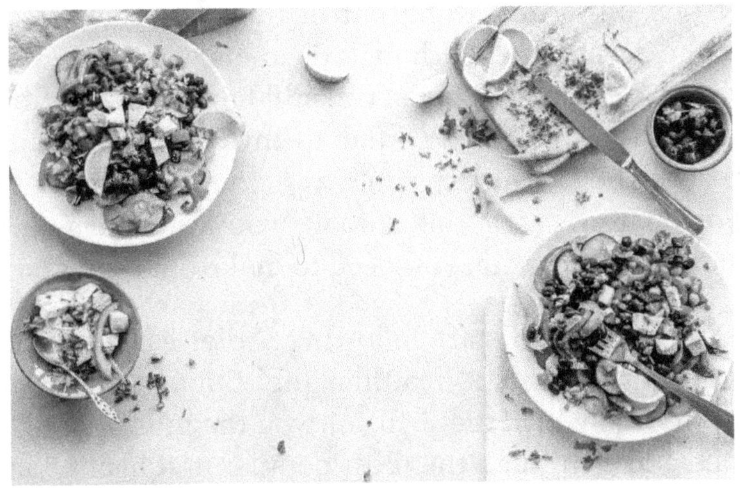

Fig. 1: Super Diets. Unsplash, by Ella Olsson, 2018, https://unsplash.com/photos/rD3YrnhTmfo/ Copyright 2018 by Ella Olsson/Unsplash.

Have you ever tried following a diet before?

These days, dieting has become very popular with different types of people and for different reasons. Some people follow diets to lose weight, some want to overcome an illness, and some just want to improve their overall health. No matter what your reason is, finding the right diet can be a huge challenge.

Along with the different diet trends that are spreading all over the world, another common phenomenon occurs with most dieters. They choose a diet (mainly because it's very popular and it promises fast results), they start following it, and when they don't see these fast results, they give up. After this process, these people find themselves back at square one feeling frustrated with themselves and with the time they "wasted" on the diet.

Is this situation familiar to you?

If so, this eBook will change things for you. Before moving on, let's get one important thing out of the way—there is no such thing as the perfect diet. Although the diets we will be discussing here are some of the best ones, you still have to determine which one is right for you. If you want to invest in your health and achieve your health goals, educating yourself is just the first step. Fortunately, with this eBook, you will learn all of the fundamental information you need to make the right choice.

Making the choice to start following a diet can potentially set you on a path towards a healthier life. But for this to happen, you need to find which diet will suit you the most. In this eBook, we will be going through the most popular and healthiest "super diets" you can follow—the Mediterranean diet, the ketogenic diet, the vegan diet, the Paleolithic diet, the flexitarian diet, and intermittent fasting. By learning the basics of these diets, you can:

- Discover what these diets are and what is involved with following each diet.
- Learn about the benefits and potential risks of each diet.
- Find out what foods you should eat and what foods you will have to avoid while following each of these diets.
- Explore the different ways to start and follow each diet.

By learning all of these things, you will have a better idea of which diet would suit your lifestyle the most. The best part is, the final chapter will help you make the best choice after you have learned about the different diets. When you are done with this eBook, you will have gained practical enlightenment from the wealth of information contained within the pages. Then all you have to do is make your choice (or at least narrow down your options) and learn more about the diet that has caught your interest.

If you're ready to learn about these super diets, now is the best time. There is no time like the present to start making a positive change in your life by making healthier dietary changes. With each chapter, you will learn something new about these super diets, whether you are a beginner or you have heard about these before. So now, let's begin your learning journey to discover the secrets of these incredible super diets!

Chapter 1:
The Mediterranean Diet

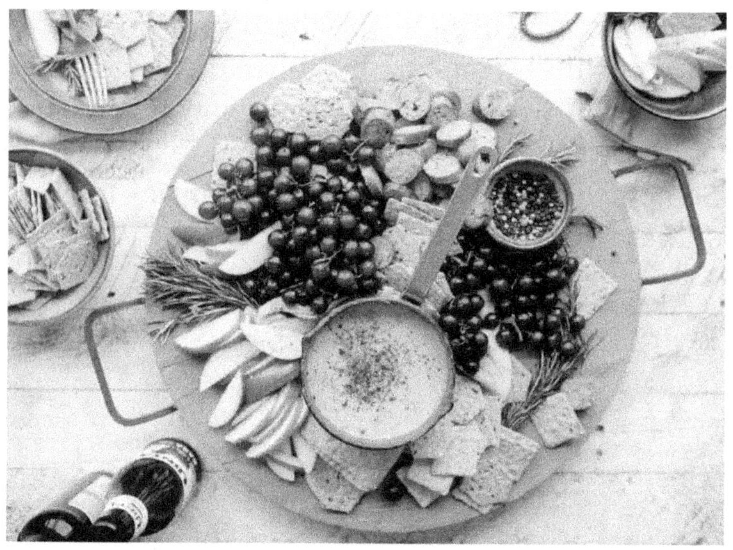

Fig. 2: Mediterranean. Unsplash, by Brooke Lark, 2017,
https://unsplash.com/photos/C1fMH2Vej8A/ Copyright 2017 by
Brooke Lark/Unsplash.

The Mediterranean diet is considered by many to be a super diet because of how unbelievably simple and healthy it is. The bases of this diet are the traditional foods eaten in Greece, Italy, and other Mediterranean countries back in the 1960s. According to researchers and health experts, the people in these countries around those times were incredibly healthy and they had a very low risk of disease, especially when compared to the American population. This diet is so effective that it has never lost its popularity over the years. The best part is this diet is easily customizable as it only comes with general guidelines and recommendations, making it perfect for you if you don't want to follow a strict diet.

What Is the Mediterranean Diet?

The Mediterranean diet is very popular, but what a lot of people don't know is that it's more of an eating pattern than a diet. Instead of following strict rules like counting calories and eliminating entire food groups, following this diet involves taking inspiration from the diets of the countries in Southern Europe. Although not entirely plant-based, this diet focuses mainly on plant foods like fresh vegetables, fresh fruits, olive oil, grains, and beans. But you can also eat other types of food like oily fish, unsaturated fats, moderate consumption of dairy products, and a low intake of meat.

By following the Mediterranean diet, you will also learn how to follow the healthy eating habits of those from Spain, Portugal, Italy, Greece, and Southern France. This diet and the healthy habits that go with it can help you achieve positive health outcomes. Aside from being a healthy diet, the Mediterranean diet offers an enjoyable way of eating. As you follow this eating pattern, you learn how to focus on good food, wonderful flavors, and taking pleasure in each of your meals.

One thing you won't see in this diet is structure. It's very easy to follow as long as you learn how to balance your meals based on the food pyramid of the Mediterranean diet. This diet pyramid helps you go on a path towards improving your long-term health. Since the Mediterranean diet is more of an eating pattern, you will have to discover how to adjust and modify it to reach your health goals. For instance, if your main health goal is to lose weight, then you have to figure out the number of calories you should consume each day to shed those excess pounds. If you have already achieved your target weight, you can modify this diet once again to help you maintain that healthy weight.

While following this diet, it would also be better for you to remain physically active. As with all other diets (yes, even the super diets), regular exercise should always be part of the equation if you want to lead a healthier, happier life. By following the Mediterranean diet that focuses on whole, healthy foods, you will start forgetting about processed and junk foods. Although you don't have to strictly eliminate these from your diet, getting used to natural foods will help you realize that you don't have to opt for the unhealthy options even though they may seem more convenient. Instead, your plate will be healthy, delicious, and bursting with vibrant colors.

The Benefits of the Mediterranean Diet

Now that you know all about the Mediterranean diet and how easy it is to follow, you might be considering it as your choice of super diet. If you're fond of natural, whole foods, then this could be the best diet for you. Apart from learning how to have healthier eating habits, you can expect the following benefits too:

Delicious, Enjoyable Meals

Since the Mediterranean diet focuses on healthy foods and flavorful meals, you will surely enjoy following this eating pattern. Even if you are currently following an "unhealthy diet," you don't have to make drastic changes. Instead, you can simply make minor changes to ensure that you're following the diet properly. For instance, if you love pizza, you can opt for one with cheese and colorful veggies instead of a pizza filled with processed meat. You can also fill your plate with fresh foods that will make you feel fuller without increasing your caloric intake too much.

Feeling Full and Satisfied

While on this diet, you will enjoy a lot of foods that are rich in healthy fats, fiber, and other satiating ingredients. This means that you will always feel full and satisfied after every meal. It also means that you can say goodbye to your cravings!

Disease Protection

This diet also encourages you to focus on plant-based foods, most of which are rich in antioxidants. These antioxidants will help protect you from various diseases while protecting your physical and mental health. By following this healthy diet, you can feel happier while gradually reducing your risk of developing health issues in the future.

Cognitive Health

Because of the nature of this diet, it can also help decrease your risk of developing brain-related issues like Alzheimer's Disease and age-related cognitive decline. Your brain is one of the hungriest organs in your body. By supplying it with sufficient energy from healthy food sources, you can maintain your cognitive health. This benefit also comes from the high antioxidant content of the foods in the Mediterranean diet.

Heart Health

You can also maintain healthy blood pressure and cholesterol levels through this diet. These effects will help reduce your risk of cardiovascular disease. The very nature of this diet makes it heart-healthy as you will see the same foods that are recommended by the American Heart Association. Since you aren't encouraged to consume processed food items on this diet, this is another eating habit that promotes the health of your heart.

Gut Health

The more you stick with this diet, the more you can nurture good bacteria in your microbiome. This benefit mainly comes from the increased intake of fruits, vegetables, and legumes.

Diabetes Prevention

This diet can also help prevent the development of type 2 diabetes. This is mainly due to the increase in your fiber intake. Since your body digests fiber at a slower rate, you won't experience significant fluctuations in your blood sugar levels. If you already suffer from this condition, the diet may help improve your diabetes markers, especially if you stick with it long-term.

Weight Loss

Although you will be focusing on oils, cheese, and nuts, this diet can potentially help you lose weight too. Since you will be consuming foods that are filling and satisfying, you won't feel hungry all the time. If you pair this diet with regular exercise and you can gradually decrease your portions, you can shed those stubborn excess pounds without feeling deprived or restricted. The best part about this benefit is that you can lose weight in a safe, healthy, and sustainable way—although not as fast as other diets. And when you have achieved a healthy weight, you can maintain it by continuing with this super diet.

Increased Longevity

With all of the benefits the Mediterranean diet has to offer, it's only natural that you will also enjoy increased longevity. Since this diet will potentially improve your overall health while protecting you from disease, you can live a happier, healthier, and longer life too. Who wouldn't want that?

Potential Risks and Side Effects

Although the proponents of the Mediterranean diet only have good things to say about it, this healthy eating pattern does come with one very significant risk. If you have a hyper-sensitive system, you may have to be careful with this diet. Having a hyper-sensitive system means that you should only consume foods that are safe for you—those which your doctor has recommended. But if you want to start following the Mediterranean diet, you should prepare for it first. Here are some tips:

- Do extensive research about the Mediterranean diet after reading this book, then make a list of all the aspects of the diet that are good and bad for you.
- Ask your doctor for a list of foods that you should eat and foods that you should avoid. Also, come up with your own lists based on your own experiences and observations. These lists will help you plan your diet later on.
- Armed with the knowledge you have gained from your research, consult with your doctor about your plan to start the Mediterranean diet. Talk about your reasons for wanting to follow the diet and any concerns you have, especially since you have a hyper-sensitive system.

Although this diet only comes with this one significant risk, some people claim that it also has its own set of downsides. Here are a few you should be aware of:

- **Increasing your mercury intake**

  If seafood wasn't part of your diet before, then this might be a concern for you. Fortunately, it's quite easy to avoid this. Try to vary your seafood sources and opt for low-mercury seafood options like salmon, tuna, catfish, and shrimp instead of mackerel, swordfish, and other seafood with high mercury content.

- **Consuming excess fats**

  Since this diet encourages you to consume healthy fats, it's very easy to go overboard. If you're not careful, you might end up consuming more fats than the recommended amount. Even if you only consume healthy fats, excess amounts still aren't good for you. So you still have to be aware of what you put on your plate.

- **Making the diet more complex than it is**

  This is probably one of the simplest diets you can follow, but some people make it more complex than it should be by imposing their own rules and restrictions. If you want to enjoy this diet and make the most out of it, stick with the general guidelines and have fun discovering your own customized version of this healthy eating pattern.

- **Limiting your milk intake**

  If you are the type of person who gets most of your calcium from milk, then this is one downside for you as you would have to limit your milk intake while on this diet. The good news is that you can get calcium from other food sources like kale, tofu, sardines, and even fortified food products like cereals and almond milk. But if you really don't want to give up milk, consider switching to skim milk.

- **Having to learn how to cook your own meals**

  Although simple, you may have to learn how to prepare and cook your own meals, especially if you want to stick with the diet long-term. If you aren't a fan of cooking or you don't have time for it, this can be a huge disadvantage for you. Of course, you can't opt for takeout or restaurant food all the time as this isn't economical.

- **Spending too much money on ingredients**

  Speaking of spending too much, if you take this diet too seriously and only opt for "traditional" Mediterranean ingredients, you will surely have to spend a lot. This is especially true if traditional ingredients aren't readily available in your local supermarkets. Also, certain fruits and vegetables are only available in specific seasons but if you really want to eat them, you would have to pay a higher price.

This is where customization comes in. You don't have to stick with traditional ingredients only, especially when you're just starting out. Instead, you can use these ingredients as inspiration and find alternatives that are readily available in your supermarkets as these would be a lot cheaper.

It's also important to note that you should still focus on moderation while following the Mediterranean diet even though it comes with few potential risks and side effects. You should also remember to include regular exercise as part of your transition to help enhance the effects and benefits of the diet. If you can overcome or even ignore these potential downsides, then this diet may truly be the one that will change your life.

Foods to Eat and Avoid

Since the Mediterranean diet focuses on healthy, whole foods, you have a wide range of options to choose from. This diet is fairly flexible because it takes inspiration from different countries, which each have their own traditional versions of the Mediterranean diet. If you want to make the most out of this diet while enjoying it in the process, finding the best foods, food combinations, dishes, and recipes is all up to you. As long as you know what foods to eat and what foods to avoid, you can easily plan your own version of this diet that will suit your lifestyle and preferences.

Foods to Eat

The menu on this diet is huge, which is one of the reasons why it's both enjoyable and sustainable. Whether you have never tried Mediterranean food before or you're already quite fond of this cuisine, you may soon become a huge fan when you discover how diverse this diet can be. Here are the foods you can eat while following the Mediterranean diet:

- **Dairy products** (in moderation) like Cheese, Greek yogurt, plain yogurt, and so on.
- **Eggs** like chicken, duck, and quail eggs.
- **Fish and seafood** like clams, crab, mackerel, mussels, oysters, salmon, sardines, shellfish, shrimp, trout, tuna, and so on. Try to have fish and seafood at least 2 to 3 times each week.
- **Fruits** like apples, apricots, bananas, dates, figs, grapes, lemons, melons, oranges, peaches, pears, strawberries, and so on. For these, you should have at least 2 servings each day.
- **Legumes** like beans, chickpeas, lentils, peas, peanuts, pulses, and so on.
- **Nuts** like almonds, cashews, hazelnuts, macadamia nuts, walnuts, and so on.
- **Poultry** like chicken, duck, turkey, and so on.
- **Seeds** like pumpkin seeds, sunflower seeds, and so on.
- **Healthy fats** like avocados, avocado oil, coconut oil, extra virgin olive oil, olives, and so on. For these, you may have up to 8 servings each day.
- **Herbs and spices** like bay leaves, basil, cilantro, cinnamon, coriander, garlic, mint, nutmeg, pepper, and rosemary, sage, and so on.
- **Tubers** like sweet potatoes, turnips, white potatoes, yams, and so on.

- **Vegetables** like broccoli, Brussels sprouts, carrots, cauliflower, cucumbers, eggplants, kale, leafy greens, onions, peppers, spinach, tomatoes, zucchini, and so on. For these, you should have between 3 to 9 servings each day.
- **Whole grains** like barley, brown rice, buckwheat, corn, rye, whole oats, whole wheat, whole-grain bread, whole-grain pasta, and so on. For these, you may have between 1 to 10 servings each day.

When it comes to beverages, your go-to option should be water. But you can also have plain coffee, plain tea, and a glass of red wine once a day. Basically, you should just try to avoid beverages that are high in sugar like sodas and processed fruit juices. You may enjoy red meat too, but not as much as the foods above.

Foods to Avoid

While the Mediterranean diet isn't as strict as other diets (yes, even the other super diets in this eBook), it does come with a number of foods that you should avoid mainly because they are considered unhealthy. Here are the foods you should try to minimize or avoid while following the Mediterranean diet:

- **Foods with added sugar** like candies, cookies, ice cream, pastries, table sugar, and so on.
- **Highly-processed food products** labeled "diet," "low-fat," or anything that looks like it came from a food factory.
- **Processed meat products** like hot dogs, sausages, and so on.
- **Refined grains** like pasta made from refined wheat, white bread, and so on.

- **Refined oils** like canola oil, cottonseed oil, palm oil, soybean oil, and so on.
- **Trans fats** found in most processed foods, margarine, and so on.

When you're starting out, you have to practice reading food labels whenever you go shopping. This allows you to check whether the foods you want to buy fit into the Mediterranean diet or not. While on this diet, you don't have to eliminate sweets altogether. If you want to satisfy your sweet tooth, you can opt for food items that are made with natural sweeteners such as honey and cinnamon.

If you have been eating a lot of the foods on this second list, then you may have to adjust to the Mediterranean diet. But the good news is, the first list—the foods to eat—is much longer, which means that you have a lot of options to choose from. And when you start feeling the good effects of this healthy diet, you will understand why these foods come highly recommended.

Tips for Starting and Following the Mediterranean Diet

Considered one of the healthiest diets in the world, the Mediterranean diet is simple, easy, and very flexible. By knowing the foods to eat and foods to avoid, you can start creating your own plan for following this diet. Although you should do your own research before following the Mediterranean diet, here are a few beginner tips to help you out:

- **Opt for olive oil when cooking**

  If you plan to start cooking your own meals (and you should!), opt for olive oil over butter, vegetable oil, or other processed oils commonly used for cooking. Olive oil is extremely healthy and nutrient-rich, making it the perfect choice for cooking on this diet. You can even use olive oil to add flavor to your dishes by drizzling it over chicken or fish. Using olive oil in salad dressings is very common too. As long as you need to add oil to a dish, opt for olive oil. While on the Mediterranean diet, this can be your main source of healthy fats.

- **Share your meals with those you love**

To make this diet more enjoyable and sustainable for you, share it with your loved ones. While you don't have to convince them to follow the same diet, share the meals that you have cooked as often as possible. This helps you transition into the diet easily while making it a more enjoyable experience for you.

- **Savor each bite**

If you really want to appreciate the foods on this diet, try to savor each bite. Instead of wolfing down everything on your plate, take your time. Sit down to eat your meals and if possible, share your meals with your family. This allows you to recognize your body's natural hunger signals which help you recognize if you're already full to avoid overeating.

- **Include veggies in every meal**

From breakfast to dinner and all meals in between, your plate should include veggies. Yes, even snacks. Vegetables are an essential part of the Mediterranean diet so if you want to succeed in it, you should start eating more of these nutrient-rich food items. The best part is, there are so many different types of veggies to choose from and you can cook them in different ways. Most of the time, you can even eat your veggies without cooking them. If you can increase your vegetable intake significantly, you can also increase the chances of experiencing all the wonderful benefits of the Mediterranean diet.

- **Increase your fish intake**

If the most abundant food on your plate should be vegetables, the most important protein source you should opt for on this diet is fish. Specifically, you should opt for mackerel, sardines, salmon, and other fatty fish. You can also opt for leaner fish as these serve as an excellent source of protein too. As with veggies, there are many different types of fish for you to choose from and you can cook them in different ways. If you eat a lot of red meat, try swapping meat with fish more often so that you can transition into this healthier eating pattern effectively.

- **Enjoy filling whole grains**

One of the things about the Mediterranean diet that a lot of people appreciate is the fact that you don't have to eliminate grains from your diet. But you should still make a change as you will have to opt for whole grains instead of the refined varieties. These are healthier, more filling, and they fit right into the Mediterranean diet.

- **Have dairy products and eggs too**

When it comes to dairy products, it's best to consume these moderately while on the Mediterranean diet. However, since there are several dairy products that are highly-processed, you must be careful when choosing what to buy. For instance, when choosing yogurt products, it's best to opt for Greek yogurt or unflavored varieties. This is why it's important to read food labels to ensure that you are only choosing the healthiest options.

Eggs are a valuable source of protein, healthy fats, and other nutrients. This makes them an amazing addition to your diet. The best part is, you can cook eggs in different ways and add them to different dishes.

- **Enjoy fruit to satisfy your sweet tooth**

Although sweets aren't recommended on this diet (you aren't prohibited from eating sweets, but it would be better if you can avoid them), you can continue eating sweet treats without feeling guilty by focusing on fruits. These healthy foods are rich in nutrients and they will easily satisfy your sweet tooth. If you're craving a sweet snack or you want something sweet for dessert, pick up a piece of fruit instead of a bar of chocolate. There are so many fruits to choose from that you will never be bored!

- **Munch on nuts for your snacks**

For filling and healthy snacks, opt for nuts. Apart from being a great addition to different types of dishes, nuts can be a tasty on-the-go snack. For instance, instead of having a plate of cookies or a bag of chips, why don't you snack on a handful of almonds? Some people are hesitant when it comes to nuts mainly because of their fat content. But most nuts contain healthy fats, which are essential for your health. Just stay away from processed nut snacks that contain excess sodium or sugar so you don't end up causing more harm to your health than good.

- **Remember... water is your friend!**

No matter what diet you are on, water will always be an essential part of it. Water is the healthiest beverage you can drink as it cleanses your body and keeps you hydrated throughout the day. Make sure that you are getting enough water each day as you start transitioning into your new, healthier diet.

- **Relax with a glass of red wine**

Wine is part of Mediterranean cuisine so this alcoholic beverage isn't completely prohibited on the diet. You can have a glass of wine each day (two glasses if you're a man) to relax and wind down after a long day's work. Sharing this glass of wine with your family while eating together is another way for you to make this diet more enjoyable and sustainable. But if you're not a fan of wine, that's okay too.

- **Say goodbye to fast foods, junk foods, and processed foods**

If these types of food are part of your current diet, then gradually eliminating them will probably be the most challenging part of your diet. Unfortunately, these foods can be so addictive and convenient, which is why most of us are fond of them. However, these foods aren't really healthy. Although you may still continue eating them, it would be more beneficial for your health to eliminate them from your diet. Instead, focus on whole, natural foods that are rich in nutrients. But if you consistently follow the Mediterranean diet, you will discover that natural foods taste better and are much more filling than fast, junk, and processed foods.

- **No need to count your calories**

  Counting calories isn't something that you have to deal with when following the Mediterranean diet. Even if you want to lose weight, you don't necessarily have to count calories. Instead, you will learn how to listen to your body, your natural signals, and make adjustments to your diet to help you reach your health goals.

As you can see, starting the Mediterranean diet is easy. You can make things interesting for yourself by eating different types of food, different types of dishes, and different types of cuisines. The longer you stick with this healthy eating pattern, the more you will discover how amazing it is and how it makes incredibly positive changes in your health.

Chapter 2:
The Ketogenic Diet

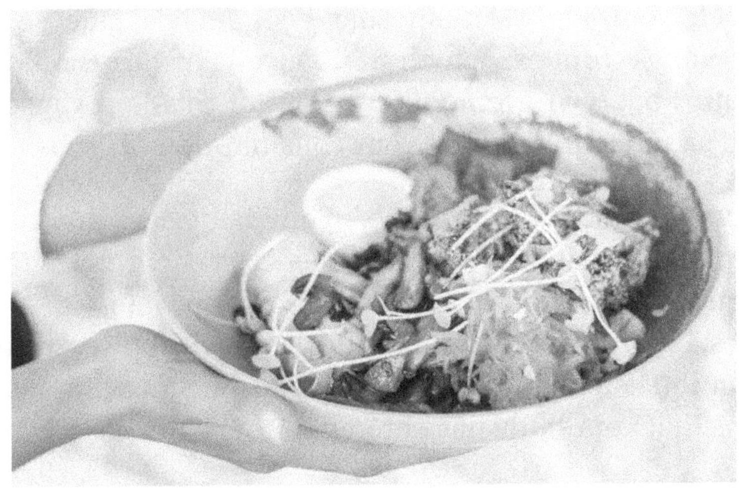

Fig. 3: Keto. Unsplash, by Maddi Bazzocco, 2018,
https://unsplash.com/photos/qKbHvzXb85A/ Copyright 2018 by
Maddi Bazzocco/Unsplash.

Another amazing super diet that is taking the world by storm is the ketogenic diet or "keto" for short. This diet has gained popularity all over the world as one of the most popular diets, especially for weight-loss. Although this diet was originally developed as part of the treatment for children with epilepsy, it has now gained followers from all walks of life. In a nutshell, the ketogenic diet is a low-carb, high-fat diet with moderate protein.

Although there are many low-carb diets out there, this has gained the top spot as the most popular because of how effective it is.

What Is the Ketogenic Diet?

The ketogenic diet involves high consumption of fat, moderate consumption of protein, and low consumption of carbs. The name "ketogenic" or "keto" comes from the fuel molecules your body produces while following this diet. While following a high-carb diet, your body's main source of fuel is glucose, which mainly comes from carbohydrates. Once you start the ketogenic diet, your body will eventually run out of this fuel source since you will significantly restrict your consumption of carbs.

While in this "starvation mode," your body will automatically look for an alternative source of fuel—this time from the healthy fats you eat. As your body breaks down fats, it produces "ketones." These are fuel molecules that will power your body while on the ketogenic diet. Once the fat-burning process starts, it means that your body has entered a state known as "ketosis."

The ketogenic diet is an excellent diet for weight loss because of how it changes your body's metabolic process. As you continue following this diet, your whole body will start burning fat all day. When your insulin level drops, the fat-burning process in your body increases dramatically, and when it runs out of fat from your meals, your body will turn to its fat stores. Essentially, your body becomes a highly efficient fat-burning machine and this is when you will start seeing yourself lose weight.

Although highly effective and beneficial, this is one of the strictest diets out there. Generally, your diet would look like this:

- You will get 60 to 75% of your daily caloric consumption from fat.
- You will get 15 to 30% of your daily caloric consumption from protein.
- You will get 5 to 10% of your daily caloric consumption from carbs.

Of course, you don't have to dive right into the diet right away. If you want to follow this diet, one of the most important tips you should keep in mind is to start gradually. Since this diet is very different from what you're used to (unless you're already following another type of low-carb diet), making drastic changes in your diet will cause a huge shock to your body along with a number of adverse side effects. Fortunately, there are different types of ketogenic diets you can follow to make it easier for you to transition into it. The different types are:

- The **cyclical ketogenic diet** involves the consumption of 70 to 75% fat, 15 to 20% protein, and 5 to 10% carbs. But for this diet, you would cycle between days where you follow the diet and days where you would increase your carb intake.
- The **high-protein ketogenic diet** involves a higher consumption of protein. Therefore, your macronutrient breakdown would be 60% fat, 35% protein, and 5% carbs.
- The **standard ketogenic diet** involves the consumption of 75% fat, 20% protein, and 5% carbs. This is the most common type of diet, but it's not ideal for beginners.

- The **targeted ketogenic diet** is similar to the standard ketogenic diet but while on it, you can increase your consumption of carbs whenever you are working out.

The Benefits of the Ketogenic Diet

The ketogenic diet shares similar benefits with other types of low-carb diets, but the main difference is that this diet is much more effective. If you're thinking about following this diet, here are some benefits you can look forward to:

Treatment for Epilepsy

Since the 1920s, the ketogenic diet has been used as part of the treatment for epilepsy, specifically in children. Although this is how the diet originated, it is now used by people of different ages and for different reasons. Thanks to the keto diet, children (and adults) who suffer from epilepsy were able to reduce their need for anti-epileptic medication without worrying about seizures. This is a wonderful benefit as it also reduced their risk of experiencing side effects from their medications. Even now, the ketogenic diet is still being used for this benefit.

Blood Sugar Control

Because of this benefit, the ketogenic diet is perfect for those who suffer from type 2 diabetes and want to manage their condition more effectively. In some cases, it can even help reverse the disease. The reason for this benefit is that the keto diet helps lower your levels of blood sugar. If you suffer from diabetes, you should definitely discuss the possibility of starting this diet with your doctor. That way, you and your doctor can come up with a plan to follow the diet safely and effectively. Even if you don't have type 2 diabetes, this is still an amazing benefit that will help you avoid a number of diseases.

Improved Disease Health Markers

Apart from type 2 diabetes, following the ketogenic diet can help you avoid other diseases since it helps improve your health markers. Just like other low-carb diets, the ketogenic diet helps improve cholesterol levels and other risk factors for heart disease. Other health markers that may improve are blood pressure levels and insulin levels, both of which may help prevent metabolic syndrome.

Enhanced Mental Performance and Energy Levels

Ketones are a more effective energy source for the brain and the other functions of the body. As long as you are in ketosis, your brain will always have fuel to keep working at optimum levels. Because of this, the diet can help improve your overall mental performance. Although you may feel a bit weak when you're first starting out, your energy levels will start picking up once your body gets used to the diet. When this happens, you will enjoy high energy levels more consistently.

Gut Health

By following the ketogenic diet, you can improve the health of your gut too. This means that you won't experience cramps or gas as frequently as you did in the past. If you suffer from IBS, this diet can help reduce the symptoms that you experience. This long-term benefit results in a calmer stomach and less pain.

Appetite Control

By nature, the ketogenic diet is very satisfying. When you eat a lot of healthy fats and protein, you won't feel hungry all the time. This means that it will become easier for you to control your appetite. The longer you stick with this diet, the more you will find that your hunger pangs and cravings are dramatically decreasing. This is a great benefit if one of your main goals for following the diet is weight loss.

Improved Physical Endurance

Since this diet can help increase your energy levels, you may notice an improvement in your physical endurance too. You can even improve this benefit by following the right type of ketogenic diet to suit your active lifestyle. For instance, the targeted ketogenic diet can be a great choice for when you work out a few times a week. On the days when you work out, you can increase your carb intake to make sure that you have enough energy to burn during the workout and recover afterward.

Weight Loss

Finally, the ketogenic diet can help you lose a lot of weight too, mainly because it will turn your body into an efficient fat-burning machine. For a lot of people, this is the most important benefit and the main reason why they have decided to follow the ketogenic diet in the first place. If you want to lose weight while improving your health, then this might be the best diet for you.

As you can see, the ketogenic diet offers a number of benefits to your health. But it is important to note that you can only experience all of these benefits if you follow the diet correctly.

Although this diet might seem simple, it is very easy to make mistakes that can potentially lead to adverse side effects. This means that if you want to go keto, make sure to follow the diet correctly.

Potential Risks and Side Effects

Beneficial as the ketogenic diet is, we cannot deny the fact that it is restrictive. If you are currently on a diet that includes a lot of carbs, going keto can be a huge challenge for you. Also, because of the nature of this diet, there are certain groups of people who shouldn't follow it. These include:

- Children, unless the diet is recommended by their pediatrician.
- Pregnant and breastfeeding women.
- People who take maintenance medications for conditions like diabetes or high blood pressure, unless the diet is recommended by your doctor.
- People who suffer from type 1 diabetes.
- People who have a history of or are currently suffering from any type of eating disorder.
- People whose gallbladder has been removed since the gallbladder aids in the digestion of fat.
- People who suffer from thyroid disease.

If you fall under any of these groups, you should think twice about starting the keto diet, especially since there are other super diets you can choose from. But if you really want to go keto, the first thing you must do is to consult with your doctor about your plans to modify your diet. This will help ensure your safety.

Even if you are at the peak of your health, the ketogenic diet still comes with a number of potential side effects you might experience when you start following it. Being aware of these side effects helps you expect and prepare for them so you don't give up on the diet prematurely:

- **Keto flu**

  This is one of the most common side effects of the ketogenic diet. A few days after starting on keto, you might experience flu-like symptoms including headaches, nausea, mental fog, and even cramps. Fortunately, the symptoms will go away after a day or two. But if you can focus on healthy keto-friendly foods as you are starting out and you always make sure that you are well-hydrated, you can potentially avoid this common side effect.

- **Weakness and low energy levels**

  Although your energy levels will eventually pick up as you stick with the diet, the first few days or weeks can be very difficult. This is especially true if you started from a high-carb diet. As you are starting with the ketogenic diet, take this time to slow down, relax, and allow your body to adjust to your new way of eating.

- **Diarrhea**

  This is one side effect that some people experience because their bodies process fats in a different way. If your body isn't able to process fat efficiently, you might end up having diarrhea because your diet will primarily consist of fat. If this occurs, you may want to consult with your doctor for how to continue with the diet or you can simply wait it out. Just make sure that you drink a lot of water so you don't get too dehydrated.

- **Keto breath**

  Although this side effect is harmless, it can be quite embarrassing. Keto breath is caused by the production of ketones—the fuel molecules produced when your body breaks down fat. Fortunately, your keto breath will go away as soon as your body adjusts to the ketogenic diet.

- **Other side effects**

  Another common downside of the ketogenic diet is that it's quite a challenge to follow because of how restrictive it is. And if you don't experience all of the benefits right away, you might lose your motivation to keep going. Other potential downsides and side effects of this diet are:

  - An increased risk of developing nutrient deficiencies.
  - An increased risk of developing kidney stones.
  - Constipation due to the lack of fiber.
  - Now knowing the "proper" fat sources may result in an increased intake of saturated and trans fats, both of which are extremely unhealthy and may increase your risk of developing various diseases.

Of course, you can always avoid these risks by learning everything that you can about the diet and planning your meals carefully. When following the ketogenic diet—or any other diet for that matter—you should always put your health and safety first. If you want to make sure that you're doing everything right, consult with your doctor and talk about your plans. Your doctor may have some excellent recommendations to add to the tips you will learn at the end of this chapter. This will help reduce your risk of experiencing these side effects while increasing your likelihood of enjoying all of the wonderful benefits of the diet.

Foods to Eat and Avoid

Even though the keto diet is considered highly restrictive, there is still a large variety of food you can eat while following it. The key to success is to know the healthiest types of keto-friendly foods to help you plan your meals from breakfast to dinner and everything in between. To help you out, let's go through the foods that are allowed and prohibited on this diet.

Foods to Eat

You may have to say goodbye to many types of foods, but you still have a lot of options to choose from. Here are the foods to eat while on keto:

- **Beverages**

  It's important to maintain proper hydration while on the ketogenic diet, especially if you want to avoid the common side effects. The best beverages to drink while on keto are:

  - Coffee (unsweetened)
  - Green tea (unsweetened)
  - Non-dairy milk alternatives
  - Protein shakes
  - Water

- **Cheese**

  Cheese is high in fat making it an excellent choice for the ketogenic diet. But if you have a high risk of heart disease, you may want to control your portions. Some examples of keto-friendly types of cheese include:

  - Blue cheese
  - Brie
  - Cheddar cheese
  - Cream cheese
  - Gouda
  - Mozzarella
  - Muenster cheese
  - Swiss cheese

- **Fish and Seafood**

  Fish and seafood are low in carbs, high in protein, and some are even excellent sources of healthy fat. If you want to meet your healthy fat goals, include a lot of fatty fish in your diet such as:

  - Albacore tuna
  - Mackerel
  - Salmon
  - Sardines
  - Trout

- **Healthy Oils**

  Since you will be focusing on healthy fats, you should know the best types of healthy oils to choose, which are:

  - Avocado oil
  - Coconut oil

- Hazelnut oil
- Olive oil
- Walnut oil

- **Low-Carb Fruits**

Sugar and carbs are huge no-no's on the ketogenic diet, but this doesn't mean that you should say goodbye to all types of fruits. Since fruits are nutritious and beneficial to health, you just have to choose wisely. Some of the best fruits to enjoy on the keto diet are:

- Avocados
- Blackberries
- Cantaloupes
- Coconut
- Lemons
- Peaches
- Raspberries
- Strawberries
- Tomatoes
- Watermelon

- **Low-Carb Dairy Products**

You don't have to say goodbye to dairy products either. As long as you know which dairy products are suitable for keto, you can continue eating these healthy food items. Besides, most dairy products are excellent sources of fat. Some examples of keto-friendly dairy options are:

- Butter
- Cream
- Greek yogurt
- Milk

- Plain yogurt

- **Low-Carb Vegetables**

Vegetables are always an important part of a healthy diet. But while you are following keto, you should stay away from starchy and high-carb veggies. Instead, focus on those which contain a lot of fiber and nutrients sans the carbs. Some examples of these are:

- Asparagus
- Bell peppers
- Broccoli
- Cauliflower
- Collard greens
- Kale
- Leafy greens
- Lettuce
- Green beans
- Spinach
- Zucchini

- **Meat, Poultry, and Eggs**

These are all healthy sources of fat and protein. When it comes to meat and poultry, opt for the fresh variety instead of processed products. As for eggs, you can cook them in different ways to keep your diet varied and interesting. Some of the best meat and poultry sources include:

- Beef
- Chicken
- Duck
- Game

- Lamb
- Pork
- Turkey
- Veal

- **Nuts and Seeds**

  These are excellent sources of protein, healthy fats, and other essential nutrients. You can add these to your dishes or have small portions of nuts and seeds for a snack. Just opt for the low-carb varieties to ensure that you don't consume excess carbs. Here are some examples of nuts and seeds for you:

  - Almonds
  - Brazil nuts
  - Cashews
  - Chia seeds
  - Flaxseeds
  - Macadamia nuts
  - Pecans
  - Pistachios
  - Pumpkin seeds
  - Sesame seeds
  - Walnuts

You can even eat dark chocolate and cocoa powder on this diet. And you can use these ingredients to create wonderful dishes that will keep you motivated to stick to the plan.

Foods to Avoid

If you decide to start following the ketogenic diet, you have to say goodbye to a number of foods and food groups. This is one reason why a lot of people find this diet too challenging to follow. Here are the foods you must avoid:

- Alcoholic beverages like cocktails and other blended varieties.
- Baked goods like bread, donuts, cakes, and croissants.
- Beans and legumes like chickpeas, kidney beans, lentils, and peas.
- Chips and other processed snack products.
- Juices, smoothies, and sodas.
- Grains and grain-based food like crackers, pasta, rice, and even beer.
- Starchy fruits like apples, bananas, grapes, oranges, pears, pineapples, and tangerines.
- Starchy vegetables like beets, carrots, corn, squash, sweet potatoes, parsnips, potatoes, and yams.
- Sweetened yogurt.
- Sugar in any form, including maple syrup and honey.
- Sugary treats like candy and ice cream.

Tips for Starting and Following the Ketogenic Diet

The ketogenic diet seems very intimidating, especially since you have to eliminate different foods and food groups from your diet. But understanding that the rules of this diet will help you transform your body into a fat-burning machine should help you see why you need to get rid of certain foods (carbs) and increase your consumption of others (fats). If you're interested in following this diet, here are some practical tips for you to start with:

- ## Ease into the diet gradually

If you want to find success on keto, don't force yourself to change your diet drastically. Instead, make small changes in your diet as time goes by to give your body and mind ample time to adjust to it. For instance, you can start by eliminating foods that you don't consume regularly anyway. Then you can move on to foods that you are eating more frequently and keep going until you have successfully transitioned into the ketogenic diet. One clever way to approach this is by making a list of foods to avoid then cross out the foods that you have already eliminated one by one until you have crossed off all the foods on your list.

- ## Choose the right type of diet

Since there are different types of keto diets you can follow, choose the one that suits your own lifestyle and health goals. You can start with the easiest type of keto diet first. When you have gotten used to it, you can level up your keto journey by choosing one of the more intense types. Learn how to listen to your body as this will tell you whether you can take things up a notch or if you should remain on the diet you are following for a few more weeks.

- ## Find the healthiest sources of fat and protein

When planning your meals, you want to focus on the healthiest sources, especially at the beginning. Since your body will be going through a number of changes, choosing healthy sources will ensure that you get all of the nutrients you need to stay healthy even if you are gradually eliminating foods from your diet.

- **Increase your water intake**

  This is an important tip, especially if you want to avoid the common side effects of the keto diet. You should always make sure that you are getting enough water all day, every day. Water helps cleanse your body, and it also keeps you hydrated so that your body continues functioning optimally as you transition into keto.

- **Clean up your environment**

  If you want to stick with keto, one of the best things you can do for yourself is to clean up your immediate environment. Start by going through your kitchen and pantry. Get rid of all non-keto-friendly foods, but don't throw them away. You can donate the food items that don't belong in your new diet or you can give them to your friends or family members who don't live in the same house as you. After this, you can start stocking your kitchen and pantry with keto-friendly ingredients and snacks. This will make it easier for you to follow the diet since you will only have keto-friendly options available at home when your hunger strikes.

- **Give meal planning a try**

  Another clever way to stick with the ketogenic diet is through meal planning. This involves planning your meals for a certain number of days—usually a week—then shopping, cooking, and preparing the meals you have planned. You would then store the meals you have prepared so that all you have to do throughout the week is heat what you have prepared. If you feel like you don't have time to cook your own keto-friendly meals every day, this is a great way to make your keto journey easier.

By setting a schedule for meal planning, you will have meals to eat for breakfast, lunch, dinner, and snacks throughout the week!

- **Make reading food labels a habit**

  Finally, make it a habit to read food labels and ingredient lists. When shopping for ingredients and snacks or even when you're eating out, make sure to read everything carefully. When you cook your own food, you know exactly what goes into each dish. But if you want to purchase keto-friendly foods, you should read the labels first to make sure that the products you buy are truly keto-friendly.

The ketogenic diet doesn't have to be difficult if you know how to follow it correctly. Soon, your body will start adjusting to the diet, and this is when you will start experiencing the many benefits that this super low-carb diet has to offer.

Chapter 3:
The Vegan Diet

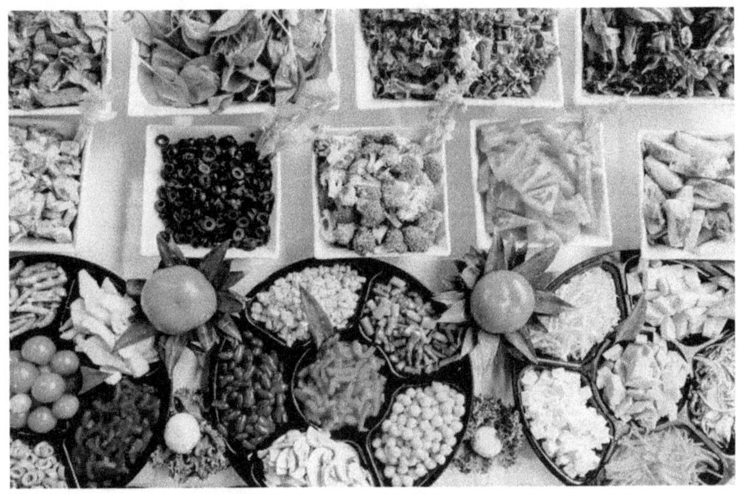

Fig. 4: Vegan. Unsplash, by Dan Gold, 2018,
https://unsplash.com/photos/4_jhDO54BYg/ Copyright 2018 by Dan
Gold/Unsplash.

For those who follow the vegan diet, it's more of a lifestyle than a simple diet. As a vegan, you won't be eating any animal-based products and you won't be using any animal-derived products either. Some vegans even avoid foods that have been processed using animal products like some types of wines and refined white sugar, for example. This is also considered a super diet because it comes with a number of health benefits. Being a plant-based diet, veganism has been in existence for quite a long time, but in recent years, it has taken the world by storm.

What Is the Vegan Diet?

These days, more and more people are becoming interested in plant-based diets, and probably the most well-known type of plant-based diet is the vegan diet. What sets this diet apart is that it goes beyond the foods you choose. Many vegans choose this diet—this lifestyle—for health, environmental, and ethical reasons. By definition, veganism is a way of living that involves the exclusion of all forms of animal cruelty and exploitation for different purposes. Therefore, when you follow the vegan diet, you will be avoiding all animal-based and animal-derived products such as eggs, dairy, and meat.

If you are thinking about following the vegan diet, you may have reasons that go beyond the improvement of your health. Whether you are also concerned about the environment or you have ethical reasons for wanting to go vegan, making this choice can initiate a huge improvement in your health since it also happens to be another super diet that offers amazing health benefits. At the beginning of your vegan journey, you may focus mainly on changing your diet. After some time, you can decide whether you want to change other aspects of your life as well wherein you will stop using household, clothing, or personal items that have been derived from animals.

Although a lot of people believe that veganism is the same as vegetarianism, these are two very different diets and lifestyles. The main difference between these two diets is that vegetarians may consume animal-derived products like eggs, dairy products, or both, while vegans do not. Just like the ketogenic diet, the vegan diet is quite restrictive. If you have been following the

Standard American Diet, transitioning to the vegan diet could be very challenging for you.

There are various types of vegan diets you can choose from depending on your health goals and your strategy for starting or following this diet. The different types are:

- The **80/10/10 vegan diet** wherein you focus on plant foods that are rich in healthy fats like avocados and nuts along with soft greens and raw fruits.
- The **junk food vegan diet** where you focus on vegan alternatives to animal-based foods like cheese, meat, and dairy along with highly-processed vegan food items. Obviously, this isn't the best option if you choose to go vegan.
- The **raw food vegan diet** wherein you only focus on raw plant foods or those which you have cooked at low temperatures (below 118°F).
- The **raw till 4 vegan diet** wherein you only consume raw foods until 4:00 in the afternoon. Then you can enjoy cooked fare for your last meal of the day.
- The **starch solution vegan diet** wherein you focus on starchy cooked plant foods like rice, corn, and potatoes rather than raw fruits.
- The **whole-food vegan diet** wherein you only focus on whole plant foods like vegetables, fruits, legumes, seeds, nuts, and whole grains.

The Benefits of the Vegan Diet

As with all the other super diets featured in this eBook, the vegan diet comes with its own benefits. No matter what your reason is for wanting to go vegan, following the diet correctly can potentially allow you to enjoy these benefits:

Nutrient-Rich

This is the most important benefit of the vegan diet. As you transition from the Standard American Diet, you will be eliminating animal-based and animal-derived products from your diet. Then you will be focusing on plant-based foods, which typically contain more nutrients. No matter what type of vegan diet you choose (except the junk food vegan diet), you will be increasing your consumption of nutrient-rich foods. Naturally, this will help increase your overall health as your body is flooded with antioxidants, vitamins, minerals, fiber, and healthy plant compounds.

Heart Health

As you focus on low-fat, high-fiber plant foods, this promotes your heart health too. This diet helps improve your health markers in relation to heart health and reduces your risk of developing heart disease.

Stable Blood Sugar Levels

Another excellent benefit you can look forward to is the stabilization of your blood sugar levels. Since plant foods are rich in fiber, your body takes a longer time to process them and break them down, and this prevents frequent fluctuations in your blood sugar levels. With this benefit, you can even lower your risk of type 2 diabetes. If you already suffer from this condition, going vegan can make it easier for you to manage it. However, since the vegan diet is very different from the typical Western diet, you should consult with your doctor first if you suffer from type 2 diabetes or any other kind of medical condition. That way, you can be sure that the change you are planning to make will be beneficial to you without compromising your health.

Improved Kidney Function

The high consumption of protein contributes to the deterioration of our kidneys. But when you consume plant proteins instead of animal proteins, this can help improve your kidney function. It can even help slow down or prevent the progression of chronic kidney diseases.

Reduced Arthritis Pain

If you suffer from certain types of arthritis that cause you pain, the vegan diet may be particularly beneficial for you. Focusing on plant-based foods can help improve your energy levels along with the general functions of your body. These benefits allow you to move more freely to help alleviate pain, morning stiffness, and the swelling of joints, all of which are common symptoms of arthritis.

Reduced Cancer Risk

Although the vegan diet won't necessarily cure cancer, it can help reduce your risk of developing this devastating disease. The main reason for this is that the vegan diet is rich in vitamins, minerals, phytochemicals, and fiber. All of these amazing nutrients have protective properties against certain types of cancer. Also, processed meat products contain a lot of carcinogenic compounds and since you will be eliminating these from your diet, you won't have to worry about their adverse effects.

Weight Loss

Weight loss is one of the most common benefits of super diets, and this also happens to be one of the main reasons why people would choose to go on diets in the first place. Typically, vegans have lower BMIs and are thinner compared to non-vegans. This is one benefit that you can enjoy, especially if you started from a high-fat or high-carb diet. By shifting to healthier, low-carb, nutrient-rich foods, you will start losing those stubborn excess pounds in no time. The best part is, you can maintain a healthy weight as long as you stick with this diet.

The vegan diet comes with some excellent health benefits and unlike other diets out there, it's not as risky since it focuses mainly on healthy, whole foods. This is another reason why proponents of this diet believe that it is the best diet ever.

Potential Risks and Side Effects

Healthy and beneficial as the vegan diet is, it has a number of downsides that you should be aware of too. Generally, these downsides are easy to avoid, especially if you plan your meals carefully and you learn everything you can about this diet. While following the vegan diet, the potential risks are:

- **Iron deficiency**

  When you shift to this plant-based diet, you should keep track of your body's iron levels. Iron is an important mineral that helps transport oxygen to the different parts of the body. However, you might not get enough iron while on the vegan diet. Specifically, you won't be able to get heme iron since you can only get this from animal sources.

Fortunately, there is another type of iron—non-heme iron—that you can get from fruits, veggies, and other plant sources. But the body doesn't absorb non-heme iron well, which is why you might still end up with an iron deficiency if you're not careful. When you don't get enough iron in your body, you could end up feeling lethargic and weak all the time.

Another dangerous risk of iron deficiency is developing a condition known as iron-deficiency anemia. This condition occurs when your body isn't producing enough red blood cells and the effects can be very serious. To avoid these risks, you can take iron supplements along with your diet. Ask your doctor about the best iron supplements that won't compromise your health as a vegan.

- **Vitamin B12 deficiency**

This is another risk that comes with the vegan diet, and if left unchecked or untreated, it can cause a number of irreversible effects. Although vitamin B12 is essential for our health, you can only get it from animal foods. The worst part is, this particular deficiency is very difficult to detect since its symptoms are very common. When you suffer from vitamin B12 deficiency, you can experience symptoms like weakness, fatigue, constipation, appetite loss, and weight loss (not the good kind).

As the deficiency progresses, you can experience balance issues, tingling or numbness of your hands or feet, and the most severe effect is the development of dementia. These are the irreversible effects that can come from this deficiency. To combat this, you should supplement your diet with a high-quality vitamin B-12 supplement. Again, it's best to consult with your doctor to find out the best supplement you can take along with your diet.

- **Not enough protein**

While not getting enough protein is another risk, it's not as bad as iron and vitamin B12 deficiencies since you can get protein from a number of plant-based sources. However, you should still make sure that the foods you eat contain enough protein since a protein deficiency can lead to inflammation, fatigue, and even hair loss. Some of the best plant-based protein sources are soy foods, legumes, nuts, seeds, and grains like quinoa.

- **Impracticality**

Since the vegan diet involves the elimination of all animal-based and animal-derived food sources, this isn't practical for everyone. For instance, if you live in a home where everyone eats meat and you're the only one who wants to go vegan, this can be very challenging. Impracticality is one of the reasons why a lot of people start following the vegan diet and then give up after a few weeks or months.

- **Other potential risks**

Then there are the potential risks that aren't very common but can still happen depending on how you follow the diet or how your body adjusts to your plant-based dietary changes. These risks include:

- o Soy proteins can sometimes cause disruptions in thyroid and estrogen levels, especially in processed form.
- o Legumes may increase your risk of developing leaky gut because of their phytate and lectin content.
- o There is a risk in consuming too many carbs while on the vegan diet and this, in turn, might lead to conditions like blood sugar dysregulation or non-alcoholic fatty liver disease, for example.
- o There is also a risk of disordered eating when you follow this diet, especially if you over-restrict yourself.

Overall, veganism is a healthy lifestyle choice. If you want to go vegan, it's important to educate yourself about this diet and lifestyle before you start. That way, you can prepare, plan, and avoid all of these potential risks by prioritizing your health.

Foods to Eat and Avoid

As someone who is interested in following the vegan diet, you might be wondering what foods you can eat and what foods you should avoid. As with any other diet, knowing this can help you prepare to start with and follow the diet long-term. Although you will be eliminating a lot of foods from your diet when you go vegan, you will still be left with a variety of choices to keep you healthy, motivated, and interested in this plant-based diet.

Foods to Eat

As a vegan, you will be focusing on plants and plant-based food sources only. Whether you will cook these or eat them raw is entirely up to you. This would depend on what type of vegan diet you will choose to follow. As a vegan, you can eat the following foods:

- **Algae** like chlorella and spirulina are excellent sources of complete protein and they even contain iodine.
- **Fermented plant foods** like miso, kimchi, seaweed, sauerkraut, kombucha, and pickles contain vitamin K2 and probiotics to improve your gut health. These food options can even boost your body's ability to absorb minerals.
- **Fruits** on a vegan diet are highly recommended and you can eat virtually any kind of fruit you get your hands on. Fruits are rich in vitamins, minerals, and nutrients to keep you healthy and strong.
- **Legumes** like peas, beans, and lentils are excellent sources of healthy plant compounds and nutrients.
- **Nutritional yeast** adds flavor to your dishes along with protein and, in some cases, vitamin B12 too.
- **Nuts** like almonds, macadamias, cashews, and walnuts contain fiber, iron, zinc, vitamin E, selenium, magnesium, and other nutrients. You can also enjoy nut butters made from these healthy food items.
- **Plant-based dairy products** like yogurt and milk will help you get enough calcium in your diet. As much as possible, opt for the calcium-fortified varieties that also contain vitamin B12 and vitamin D.
- **Plant-based natural sweeteners** like agave, maple syrup, and coconut sugar allow you to enjoy desserts and sweet treats as a vegan. However, honey doesn't qualify as a vegan-friendly sweetener.
- **Plant-based oils and healthy fats** are suitable for the vegan diet too. If you're looking for such products, opt for cold-pressed varieties whenever possible.

- **Seeds** like chia seeds, flaxseeds, and hemp seeds contain omega-3 fatty acids and are a good protein source too.
- **Soy products** like tempeh, seitan (a meat substitute made of hydrated wheat gluten), and tofu. Adding these to your diet will boost your protein intake and give you versatility in your dishes.
- **Whole grains** like quinoa, spelt, farro, barley, and amaranth provide you with protein, iron, fiber, B-vitamins, complex carbs, and other minerals.
- **Vegetables**, especially leafy greens like spinach, bok choy, watercress, and kale are high in calcium, iron, and other essential nutrients that your body needs to survive on this plant-based diet.

These days, there are also endless varieties of vegan-friendly versions of common food items. For instance, there is vegan-friendly mayonnaise, ice cream, hot dogs, burgers, and more. Although it's best to opt for whole, natural foods while you follow the vegan diet, having these vegan-friendly alternatives once in a while can make your transition into veganism a lot easier.

Foods to Avoid

As a vegan, you have to stay away from any foods made from, derived from, or based on animals. This narrows down your food options significantly, especially if you started from the Standard American Diet. When you decide to go vegan, you have to say goodbye to these foods:

- **Animal oils and animal-based fats** like lard and fish oil.
- **Bee products** like royal jelly, bee pollen, and honey.

- **Dairy products** like butter, yogurt, cheese, milk, and ice cream.
- **Eggs** from quails, chickens, fish, and ducks.
- **Fish** such as salmon, anchovies, tuna, mackerel, and bass.
- **Meat** such as pork, lamb, beef, veal, game, and organ meats.
- **Poultry** such as duck, chicken, turkey, and quail.
- **Seafood** such as squid, crab, shrimp, lobster, scallops, and clams.

When it comes to choosing vegan-friendly foods, you have to be very careful. There are some food products that might seem to fit into this diet but when you inspect the ingredient list, you'll discover ingredients that aren't vegan friendly. Here are some examples:

- Some **baked goods and pastries** may contain egg yolks, honey, or even egg wash to give them a glossy surface.
- **Marshmallows, Jell-O, and gummy candies** may contain gelatin, which is made from the bones and skin of animals.
- **Refined white sugar** is made using animal bone char, which isn't vegan.
- Store-bought **sauces, dressings, and condiments** may contain a number of animal-based ingredients.

To make sure that you are only eating vegan-friendly fare, you should learn how to read ingredient lists, especially if you opt for store-bought food products.

Tips for Starting and Following the Vegan Diet

No matter how different the vegan diet is from your current diet, there are always ways for you to transition smoothly into it. Veganism is one of the most popular diets around the world simply because it's healthier and it promotes the consumption of natural, plant-based foods. Here are some tips for you to make it easy for you to start following the vegan diet:

- **Prepare for your vegan journey**

  Now that you know more about the vegan diet, you have a better idea of whether it's the right diet for you or not. If you think that you can thrive on this diet, you should add to your knowledge by researching it. Learning everything that you can about the vegan diet helps you understand what it's truly about. This will also help you prepare for your journey into a plant-based lifestyle.

- **Fill your plate with veggies**

  Since veganism focuses on plant-based foods, vegetables should be the star of your meals. From breakfast to dinner, pile your plate with veggies of different colors, both cooked or raw. These will make you feel full while providing you with the essential nutrients you need to improve your health.

- **Start with familiar food, then try to be more adventurous**

  Going vegan doesn't have to be a drastic change. You can start with vegan-friendly dishes like salads and vegetable stews just to make you feel comfortable with the diet.

Then you can gradually introduce new foods into your diet while you also eliminate non-vegan food options.

As you get used to the vegan diet, you can start becoming more adventurous. For instance, if you have never tried fermented foods before, you can give them a try. Who knows? You might discover some vegan food items or dishes that will end up becoming your favorites! Also, being an adventurous eater on the vegan diet will make things more interesting for you in the long-run.

- **Diversify your diet**

Another way to keep you motivated to stick with the diet is by finding ways to diversify it. Think about it: If you only eat salads at every meal, you will definitely get bored with the vegan diet after a few days or weeks. But if you learn how to cook different types of vegan dishes or try out different types of vegan cuisines, this diet will become much more interesting and appealing. Diversifying your diet also allows you to find a healthy, balanced way of eating.

- **Find vegan-friendly alternatives and substitutes**

This is one tip that can make it easier for you to transition into the vegan diet. These days, you can find vegan-friendly alternatives and substitutes for almost everything. For instance, there are vegan-friendly mock meats that you can use to make burgers. You can also make cheesy dishes using vegan-friendly cheese substitutes. There is even such a thing as vegan bacon!

One of the reasons why you should do research before jumping into the vegan diet is that you will discover these food items and products that will allow you to satisfy your non-vegan cravings without breaking your diet.

- **Take the right supplements**

As you have already learned, the biggest risks associated with the vegan diet are nutrient deficiencies. Although you can get the vitamins and minerals you need from plant-based sources, you can reduce your risk of developing deficiencies by taking the right supplements. When considering supplements to take while on this diet, some of the most important options are omega-3, iron, vitamin B12, and vitamin D. Just remember to speak with your doctor first before you start taking any kind of supplements, especially if you are also starting to follow the vegan diet.

- **Learn how to be kinder to yourself**

Veganism is more than just a diet—it's a lifestyle that teaches you to make healthier and more ethical choices. While choosing plant-based food over animal-based options shows that you care for animals, you should also learn how to care for yourself. The best way to do this is by learning how to be kind to yourself. As you start with the vegan diet, don't be too hard or too harsh on yourself. If you slip up once in a while, that's okay. Just keep trying. You will get used to the diet eventually and if you can do it without giving yourself a hard time, your vegan journey will be more fulfilling.

- **Seek support**

Finally, you can make your transition easier by finding and joining a vegan community. This allows you to learn more about veganism, feel motivated, share stories, and discover how to overcome the common challenges of going vegan. You can even go online and join forums or social media groups to talk about your journey and connect with like-minded people.

As you transition into veganism, it's also a good idea to share your vegan dishes with the other people in your home. This makes your vegan diet a more positive experience as you get to show your loved ones that this diet is far from boring. Maybe you can even convince them to start their own vegan journeys too!

Chapter 4:
The Paleolithic Diet

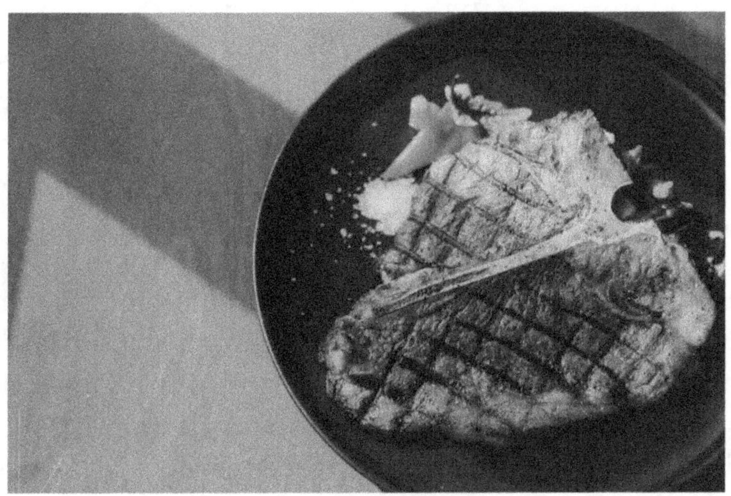

Fig. 5: Paleo. Unsplash, by Hanxiao, 2020, https://unsplash.com/photos/aLHhsDbj1Iw/ Copyright 2020 by Hanxiao/Unsplash.

The Paleolithic diet—paleo for short—is a dietary plan that focuses on foods that our ancestors would have eaten back in the Paleolithic era. Generally, this diet includes meat, fish, vegetables, fruits, seeds, and nuts. Basically, any food that could have been obtained through hunting and foraging. This diet will bring you back to the basics as you will say goodbye to the convenient, readily-available, and highly-processed foods that you can find in restaurants, supermarkets, and food shops. Since these foods are unhealthy anyway, the paleo diet is considered a super diet because it encourages you to focus on natural, whole foods to improve your health and give you a number of wonderful benefits too.

What Is the Paleolithic Diet?

The Paleo diet is one of the simplest diets out there since its core concept is very basic. While on the Paleo diet, you simply avoid all foods that cavemen didn't eat. This primitive diet is all about the foods that were available before the pre-agricultural revolution when people started making, planting, and inventing food. Before this time, our early ancestors only ate poultry, fish, meat, fruits, vegetables, and other things that they hunted and foraged.

The idea behind this diet is that the elimination of modern-day food can improve your health while helping you avoid disease. After all, it seems like our ancestors used to live longer lives, or at least, they didn't die because they got sick from the food they ate. Simple as the Paleo diet is, there is no standard way to follow it. This diet comes with a number of rules and guidelines for what to eat and avoid. But it is up to you how you will follow the diet and what types of food you will eat.

Because of the modern advancements in the food industry, we cannot really consume exactly the same foods as our hunter-gatherer ancestors ate back in the Paleolithic era. Even meats, fruits, and veggies aren't as "natural" and "wholesome" as they were in the past. If you want to go Paleo, you have to settle for a diet that closely resembles the diet followed by ancient man. You don't have to hunt and forage, but you can choose what you eat carefully.

By following the Paleo diet and pairing this with an active lifestyle, you can potentially experience a number of health benefits while reducing your risk of diseases. Aside from being one of the super diets, the Paleo diet also happens to be one of the most popular diets today. Over the years, this diet has evolved, and now, people follow different versions of it. For instance, some people don't stick rigidly with this diet. Such people include processed foods that are considered healthy. As you start following this diet, you can do this too. But if you really want to go fully Paleo, this would involve a lot of discipline as you make a number of changes in your current diet and eating habits.

The Benefits of the Paleolithic Diet

Although some people consider the Paleo diet to be too extreme, it has still risen as one of the most popular—and healthiest— diets all over the world. As you follow this diet, you will start seeing a number of changes happening in your body. In terms of benefits, the Paleo diet offers the following:

Cleaner Diet

Since the Paleo diet encourages you to focus on whole and natural foods, following it will result in a cleaner diet. You will be saying goodbye to chemicals, preservatives, additives, and other unnatural ingredients that are commonly found in processed foods. This is the most significant benefit of the diet as it will improve your overall health.

Blood Pressure Regulation

By following this diet, you may experience some improvement in your blood pressure levels. This is very beneficial, especially if you want to avoid chronic diseases like diabetes, metabolic syndrome, and heart disease.

Anti-Inflammatory Properties

The Paleo diet also offers anti-inflammatory benefits, especially if you focus on fruits, veggies, nuts, seeds, and healthy oils.

More Nutrients

When you follow this diet properly, you will consume more nutrients compared to a diet that includes too many processed foods. Here are some examples of nutrients you can get on Paleo:

- Red meat is an excellent source of iron.
- Healthy fats from olive oil and avocado can give you a healthier lipid profile.
- Fruits and vegetables are excellent sources of potassium to help maintain healthy muscle function, kidney function, and healthy blood pressure levels.

Of course, you can get even more vitamins, minerals, and nutrients from this diet if you choose the food you eat carefully. The more you focus on natural foods, the healthier you can become.

Appetite Reduction

The foods that you eat while on this diet are more filling. Since you will be focusing on healthy fats and proteins, you will always feel full and satisfied after every meal. When this happens, you will notice a reduction in your appetite and food cravings.

Weight Loss

Because of the previous benefit, you may also experience significant weight loss when you go Paleo. Another reason why you may lose weight is that you will be eliminating processed carbs from your diet. You will no longer be eating all of the empty calories that come from processed foods like potato chips, cookies, sweets, sugary beverages, and more. If weight loss isn't one of your health goals, you can at least maintain a healthy weight while on Paleo.

The benefits of Paleo are within your reach. But if you're starting to think that this is the right diet for you, it's also important to know the other side of the coin. Knowing the good and bad sides of these super diets allows you to make an informed decision on which of these will suit your lifestyle and help you achieve all of your long-term health goals.

Potential Risks and Side Effects

Unlike many other diets, the Paleo diet encourages you to eat more meat. However, this doesn't mean that you should use this as an excuse to eat too much meat without balancing it with fruits, veggies, and other whole foods. This is the biggest risk of the Paleo diet. Many people feel so excited about the prospect of eating a lot of meat that it is the only thing that they focus on.

Unfortunately, doing this won't give you the benefits discussed in the previous section. Instead, you might experience a number of adverse effects like an increase in your risk of heart disease or an elevation of your blood cholesterol levels. Apart from the risk of eating too much meat, the Paleo diet also has the following potential downsides:

- When you eliminate foods and food groups from your diet, you run the risk of missing out on essential nutrients.
- Eliminating whole grains from your diet might affect your gut health as you won't be consuming enough fiber. Your gut health might suffer too because you will also avoid legumes.
- There is a risk of exceeding the recommended daily allowances for certain types of foods.
- You might not get enough calcium, especially if you primarily get your calcium from processed foods like yogurt, milk, and cheese. This might put you at risk for low tooth and bone density.
- Most of the foods that our ancestors used to eat aren't available now. This means that we aren't really following the "authentic" Paleo diet. But if you can find foods that closely resemble those our ancestors used to eat, this doesn't have to be an issue.
- Those who have given up on the diet claim that it's too difficult and too expensive. There may be some truth to this unless you find shops in your locale where you can find fresh ingredients. If you learn how to prepare and cook your meals, the Paleo diet doesn't have to be expensive or challenging.
- If you start as a vegan, this diet might not be the best choice for you as it includes meat.

Finally, although our ancestors in the Paleolithic era may have adapted to this diet, our bodies now aren't genetically identical to theirs. Through the years, we have evolved, which means that our nutritional needs may have evolved too. However, since this diet encourages natural foods, its potential is still evident. The key to avoiding all of these risks and downsides is to know what you should eat, what you should avoid, and what supplements to take to avoid any nutrient deficiencies.

Foods to Eat and Avoid

If you choose to go Paleo, you should know what foods you can eat and which ones you should stay away from. As with any other diet, knowing the foods to eat and avoid is key. Also, having this information can help you determine if the Paleo diet is right for you or if you need to keep looking for the best super diet for you.

Foods to Eat

When choosing foods to eat while on Paleo, you should focus on whole, unprocessed options. This is the first thing you should get used to. Go around your locale to find out where you can get the following foods:

- **Eggs**

  Eggs contain protein, antioxidants, B-vitamins, and minerals. Opt for cage-free and organic eggs whenever possible. The best thing about eggs is that you can cook them in different ways to help make your diet more interesting.

- **Fruits**

Fruits are rich in fiber, vitamins, minerals, antioxidants, and other healthy nutrients. The best part is, fruits are naturally sweet. Since you should generally avoid sweet foods on this diet, fruits can help satisfy your sweet tooth. Just try to limit your consumption of fruits that are too sweet or starchy to avoid any adverse side effects. Some examples of fruits to eat on this diet include:

- Apples
- Avocados
- Bananas
- Berries like blueberries, blackberries, and raspberries
- Citrus fruits like grapefruits, lemons, and oranges
- Grapes
- Melons
- Peaches
- Plums

- **Healthy Fats and Oils**

When it comes to fats and oils, you have to be very picky because a lot of the fats and oils available are heavily processed. Opt for natural plant-based oils as these have been extracted directly from plants. Some examples of healthy fats and oils to eat on this diet include:

- Avocado oil
- Coconut oil
- Flaxseed oil
- Macadamia oil
- Olive oil
- Walnut oil

- **Meat**

Meat is an excellent source of protein to make you feel full while helping your body build and repair tissues and cells. Opt for fresh and organic meat as much as possible. Some examples of meat to eat on this diet include:

  - Bacon
  - Beef
  - Chicken
  - Duck
  - Lamb
  - Pork
  - Turkey
  - Veal
  - Wild game like bison, venison, and quail

- **Nuts and Seeds**

These are chock-full of fiber, protein, and healthy fats. Nuts and seeds belong in the Paleo diet because our early ancestors used to forage for these in nature. You can have nuts and seeds for your snacks or use them in different dishes. Some examples of nuts and seeds to eat on this diet include:

  - Almonds
  - Brazil nuts
  - Cashews
  - Chia seeds
  - Flax seeds
  - Hazelnuts
  - Macadamia nuts
  - Pecans
  - Pine nuts

- Pistachios
- Pumpkin seeds
- Sunflower seeds
- Walnuts

- **Seafood**

Seafood is also rich in protein, low in carbs, and may even contain omega-3 fatty acids. When choosing seafood, make sure it's fresh and try to opt for wild-caught as much as possible. Some examples of seafood to eat on this diet include:

- Cod
- Crab
- Mackerel
- Salmon
- Sardines
- Scallops
- Shellfish
- Shrimp
- Tuna

- **Vegetables**

Veggies are some of the most nutritious foods you can include on your diet. Unlike fruits, there are very few veggies that are high in sugar and starch. This means that you can eat as many veggies as you want. If you can, opt for organic veggies as much as possible as these don't contain as many pesticides and chemicals as non-organic varieties. Some examples of vegetables to eat on this diet include:

- Asparagus
- Broccoli
- Brussels sprouts
- Butternut squash
- Cabbage
- Carrots
- Cauliflower
- Kale
- Onions
- Peppers
- Pumpkin
- Spinach
- Sweet potatoes
- Tomatoes

When cooking your Paleo meals, you can use herbs and spices like garlic, rosemary, sea salt, and more to make your dishes healthier and more flavorful. When it comes to beverages, your go-to drink should be water. But you can also drink plain coffee and tea without milk and sugar.

Foods to Avoid

Now that you know what foods you can eat while on Paleo, you should also know what foods you should avoid. This will make it easier for you to follow the diet correctly by planning the ingredients to buy, the meals to cook, and the foods you should gradually eliminate from your current diet.

- **Artificial sweeteners** like cyclamates, aspartame, saccharin, sucralose, and acesulfame potassium.
- **Dairy products** like cheese, butter, milk, and low-fat options.
- **Grains** like pasta, bread, barley, rye, and wheat.

- **Legumes** like lentils, beans, peas, and peanuts.
- **Processed meat products** like deli meat, hot dogs, and some types of bacon.
- **Sugary foods** like baked goods, sweets, ice cream, sodas, and fruit juices.
- **Trans fats** like those found in different types of processed foods. Usually, trans fats are called "partially hydrogenated" or "hydrogenated" oils.
- **Vegetable oils** like cottonseed oil, safflower oil, soybean oil, corn oil, sunflower oil, and grapeseed oil.

Now that you know all of the foods to eat and avoid while on Paleo, you should already have an idea of whether this diet is right for you or not. If you think that it has potential, then the next thing you should learn is how you can start following it.

Tips for Starting and Following the Paleolithic Diet

For some people, transitioning to the Paleo diet is super easy but for others, it is extremely challenging. This depends on where you started and how different your current diet is from Paleo. But if you want to make your Paleo journey as smooth and easy as possible, there are things you can do. Here are some tips for you:

- **Find your motivation**

  Before you start following the Paleo diet, think about your reason for wanting to do so. Go back to the potential benefits of this diet and see if any of those appeal to you. Some of the more common reasons for following this diet is to lose weight and help overcome medical issues like allergies, GI problems, and autoimmune conditions, for example. If you know your reason (or reasons) for following this diet, it becomes easier for you to stay motivated and keep going.

- **Do your research**

This is very important, especially if you want to avoid the common risks or side effects of the Paleo diet. For instance, if you want to avoid nutrient deficiencies, research the best sources of the essential nutrients you need to stay healthy. By learning everything you can about the Paleo diet, you can follow it correctly. This will increase your chances of enjoying the benefits this diet has to offer while reducing your risk of experiencing any adverse side effects.

- **Start with a "shadow week" before diving into Paleo**

This clever method can help you transition easily into the diet. To perform your shadow week, simply eat normally for the whole week. Each time you eat, make a note of what you are eating and what is the best Paleo alternative you can eat instead. For instance, if you had a light lunch where you only ate a peanut butter and jelly sandwich, a Paleo-friendly alternative to this would be a salad with avocado, chicken, and olive oil-based dressing. You can do 1 to 2 shadow weeks to give you an idea of what Paleo meals look like and what ingredients you need to make them.

- **Continue with the 85/15 rule**

When you're done with your shadow week, you can start easing into the Paleo diet. For your first month, you can try the 85/15 rule wherein you would follow the diet strictly 85% of the time and then allow yourself to consume non-Paleo food options 15% of the time. This is a great way for you to get used to the diet without feeling too restricted. As you get used to the diet, you can gradually eliminate the non-Paleo options until you have transitioned completely.

- **Expect setbacks and challenges**

At some point, you will feel tempted to go back to your "normal diet." No matter how hard you try, there might be days when you give in to this temptation. When such a thing happens, it doesn't mean that you have failed. Such situations are simply setbacks and challenges that can happen to anyone. If you expect these things to happen, you can accept them more easily. Forgive yourself, then go back to the changes you are trying to make to your diet.

- **Learn how to "decode" food labels**

Making it a habit to read food labels is very helpful. But beyond that, you should learn how to understand the information on these labels. If you really want to avoid non-Paleo foods, you must learn how to spot non-Paleo ingredients in various food products. Practice this every time you go to the supermarket. Familiarize yourself with Paleo-friendly foods and foods you should avoid. Then try to identify all of the ingredients on food labels to see if certain products fit into your diet or not.

- **Increase your meat intake the right way**

  Since meat is an important part of the Paleo diet, you have to get used to eating meat. However, you must make sure that you are eating meat the right way. This means focusing on fresh meat, organic meat, lean meat, and pasture-fed meat options instead of processed meat products like salami, hot dogs, and other deli meats.

- **Give in to your sweet cravings**

  One of the biggest challenges beginner Paleo dieters face is eliminating sugar from their diets. The good news is, you don't have to do this. You still have the option to eat sweet treats in the form of nature's candy—fruits! If you have a craving for something sweet, give in to this craving by munching on a piece of fresh fruit instead of restricting yourself because sweets aren't recommended.

- **Cook your own Paleo-friendly meals and snacks**

  As with most diets, you can make things easier for yourself by learning how to whip up your own Paleo-friendly meals and snacks. In the long-run, this is more economical and it will keep you motivated to stick to your goals. Although buying ready-made foods is the more convenient option, this diet is more sustainable if you opt for homemade meals and snacks.

- **Commit to the diet while maintaining some level of flexibility**

  This means that you make a commitment to following the diet but you aren't too strict or too hard on yourself. If you want to follow the Paleo diet for the foreseeable future, make it a positive experience. Try different things, experiment with different foods, and keep making adjustments to your diet until you find the sweet spot where you are enjoying Paleo without breaking any rules.

Chapter 5:
The Flexitarian Diet

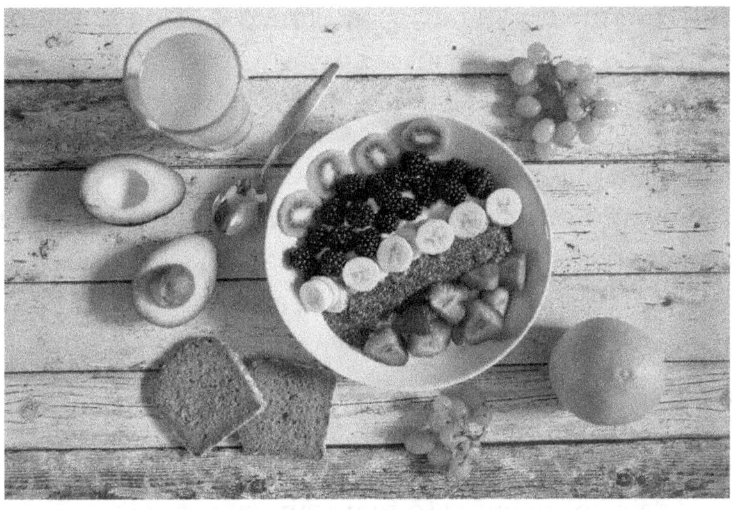

Fig. 6: Flexitarian. Unsplash, by Jannis Brandt, 2016,
https://unsplash.com/photos/8manzosDSGM/ Copyright 2016 by
Jannis Brandt/Unsplash.

Among all of the super diets we have here, this is one that some people might not be familiar with. The term "flexitarian" is a combination of the terms "flexible" and "vegetarian." This makes it a more flexible and easier approach to becoming a vegetarian. Essentially, you can still get all of the benefits of the vegetarian diet without following its strict rules. This is another healthy diet that offers simplicity, easy maintenance, and a clean approach to food.

What Is the Flexitarian Diet?

If you want to focus more on plant-based foods but you don't think that you can give up animal-based foods completely, then the flexitarian diet might be the right choice for you. The main idea behind this diet is that you can enjoy the benefits of plant-based diets (specifically the vegetarian diet) while allowing yourself to eat meat whenever you crave it. This is a simple diet that doesn't feel restrictive in any way because of the flexible aspect.

To succeed in the flexitarian diet, you should focus on plant-based meals and only allow yourself to eat meat in moderation. The plant-based foods found in the vegetarian diet are satisfying and delicious. But when your meat cravings strike, it can be very difficult to continue eating veggie dishes while feeling completely satisfied. Fortunately, this diet allows you to give in to those cravings. The best part about this diet is that you won't have to stop eating any type of food completely. All you have to do is find the right balance to maintain your health.

Some people consider the flexitarian diet as a "semi-vegetarian" diet. While on it, you can look forward to the benefits of plant-based foods without transitioning to a plant-based lifestyle completely. When you follow this diet, you focus more on the plant foods that you will incorporate into your diet instead of the animal-based foods that you will remove from it. You will be getting most of your daily caloric intake from plant sources like fruits, vegetables, whole grains, and legumes. In terms of protein, it's also recommended to focus more on plant proteins while allowing yourself to consume a moderate amount of animal proteins. As with all the other diets on our list of super diets, it's recommended to limit your intake of sweets while on the flexitarian diet.

As the name implies, this is a very flexible diet. However, this doesn't mean that you won't have to follow any rules while on it. After all, it wouldn't be considered a diet if it didn't come with some basic guidelines and recommendations. For now, let's take a look at some of these recommended guidelines to give you a better idea of what the flexitarian diet may look like:

- As a **beginner** on the flexitarian diet, you would be consuming at least 6 to 8 fully plant-based meals each week.
- As you move on to the more **advanced** stage of the flexitarian diet, you would be consuming at least 9 to 14 fully plant-based meals each week.
- As an **expert** on the flexitarian diet, you would be consuming at least 15 or more fully plant-based meals each week.

This means that the longer you stick with the diet, the more you will train yourself to focus on meatless meals.

The Benefits of the Flexitarian Diet

Since this diet is "semi-vegetarian," it potentially offers the same benefits as the vegetarian diet. As you have already learned in Chapter 3, the vegetarian diet differs from the vegan diet since the vegan diet doesn't include any animal-based foods like eggs and dairy. The flexitarian diet is even less strict as it allows you to eat meat once in a while. By following this diet, you can look forward to these benefits:

Ease and Flexibility

Naturally, the biggest benefit of this diet is the superb flexibility it offers. Although primarily plant-based, you won't have to eliminate any foods from your current diet when you follow the flexitarian diet. All you would have to do is make some adjustments to your current diet so that you consume more plant foods to make yourself healthier. The simplicity of this diet and its lack of rigidity makes it very easy and convenient to follow too.

Filling and Nourishing

Fiber is one of the main components of this diet because it includes a lot of plant sources. Because of this, the meals you eat will be more filling and satisfying. As you consume fruits, veggies, and plant-based proteins, you will end each meal feeling fuller for a longer time. Also, foods that fit into this diet are generally rich in nutrients. This means that they will nourish your body well. Plant-based foods are also rich in vitamins, minerals, and essential nutrients that will make you healthier and help you avoid a number of diseases.

Reduced Heart Disease Risk

Speaking of avoiding diseases, following the flexitarian diet can help lower your risk of stroke and heart disease. Again, this benefit comes from the fact that you will be focusing mainly on plant foods, which are generally healthier than animal-based or processed foods. Following this diet can even help treat and prevent heart failure.

Improved Insulin Resistance

Since this diet also recommends that you reduce your sugar intake, you may experience an improvement in your insulin resistance. The reduction of sugar and the increase of healthy, whole foods will help stabilize your blood sugar levels. Ultimately, this can help reduce your risk of developing type 2 diabetes. If you already suffer from this condition, following the flexitarian diet may help you manage type 2 diabetes more effectively.

Affordability

Another great benefit of this diet is that it's very economical. Since it's not considered a specialized diet and you don't have to make drastic changes to your current diet, you won't have to spend more on the food you eat. Making small changes to your diet allows you to find cheap but healthy alternatives to the foods that you will eat less of. Also, fruits, veggies, and other plant foods are generally cheaper than meats and processed foods. So if you focus on these healthy foods, you'll discover that it's a lot lighter on your wallet too.

Weight Loss

As you think about your health goals when trying to determine which diet to choose, weight loss might be at the top of your list. Fortunately, the flexitarian diet offers this benefit as well. Since the foods you will eat on this diet are more filling and satisfying, you will be able to control your appetite better. As you get used to this diet, you might also notice that you don't crave unhealthy foods as strongly as you used to. If you keep sticking with the healthy, balanced eating recommended by this diet, you may start losing weight too.

Improved Longevity

With all of the amazing health benefits this diet has to offer, you can even live longer while following it. Unlike people who follow the Standard American Diet which is full of processed, sugary, and junk foods, focusing on healthy plants and high-quality meats will improve your longevity. Since this diet helps reduce your risk of diseases, this also promotes this specific benefit. So if you want to follow a relatively easy diet that can potentially improve your health, the flexitarian diet may be the best option for you.

Potential Risks and Side Effects

Since this diet promotes balance and variety without eliminating any foods or food groups, it is generally healthy and safe for most people. But there are two groups of people who may need to be extra careful when following the flexitarian diet:

- **Pregnant women** should be very careful when following any kind of diet, even one as flexible as the flexitarian diet. Since the bodies of women undergo a number of changes throughout the pregnancy, they may need more vitamins, minerals, and nutrients. For instance, low levels of iron are very common in pregnant women. Therefore, they may have to eat more than moderate amounts of meat. Otherwise, they should ask their doctor about taking an iron supplement or any other kind of supplement to ensure their health and the health of the developing baby in their womb.

- **People with diabetes** must be careful too. Although this diet can be beneficial for those who suffer from type 2 diabetes, those who suffer from either type 1 or type 2 diabetes should be mindful of what they eat. Since many vegetarian foods have higher carb proportions, it's easy to overeat carbs. Of course, this isn't good for those who suffer from diabetes as excess carbs can have a negative effect on their blood sugar levels.

Even if you're at the peak of your health, the flexitarian diet comes with a few potential risks and downsides that you must be aware of. These include:

- **Not getting enough iron**

  Since you will be decreasing your meat intake, this may result in lower iron levels. If left unchecked, you might even suffer from iron deficiency or anemia. If you want to avoid this, you should make sure that your diet includes iron-rich plant sources like lentils, leafy greens, whole grains, seeds, and beans.

- **Challenging for those who love eating meat**

  If you're a huge fan of meat and you can't get enough of it, this diet might be too challenging for you. Although you don't have to eliminate meat from your diet completely, you would still have to reduce your consumption of this protein-rich food source. But you can easily overcome this issue by easing into the diet gradually to give your body a chance to get used to plant-based foods.

- **Risk of developing restrictive eating patterns**

  Finally, although this diet isn't restrictive in the least, there is still a risk of developing restrictive eating patterns. This typically happens if you have a history of or you are currently suffering from an eating disorder. In such a case, it's not a good idea to start a new diet, even one as simple and flexible as the flexitarian diet. Instead, you should consult with your doctor to ask for advice on how you can improve your diet and focus on healthier foods like plant-based sources. Remember that your health and safety should be your main priorities. So it's best to avoid all things labeled as "diet" so you don't end up exacerbating your disordered or restrictive eating patterns.

Foods to Eat and Avoid

The main thing that sets this diet apart from the rest is the fact that you don't have to "avoid" certain foods and food groups. Instead, you would only minimize your consumption of certain foods to help you reach your health goals.

Foods to Eat

By nature, the flexitarian diet is very simple because you are allowed to eat virtually anything on it. As you follow this diet, you will learn how to clean up your plate by filling it with plant foods, which are generally healthier and more satisfying. Here are the foods to focus on while you follow the flexitarian diet:

- **Dairy products**

  You can enjoy various dairy products while on this diet. These foods offer calcium, vitamin D, and protein too.

- **Eggs**

  These are excellent protein sources. Eggs also contain additional nutrients for a healthy, balanced diet.

- **Fruits**

  Although you technically don't have to eliminate sugar and sweets from your diet, you may want to opt for fruits if you're craving a sweet treat. Aside from satisfying your sweet tooth, fruits like avocados, apples, berries, grapes, oranges, and cherries will also nourish your body as they contain vitamins, minerals, fiber, and water.

- **Herbs, spices, and healthy oils**

  These amazing food options will add flavor and nutrients to your meals. Make your dishes more interesting by adding herbs and spices like basil, mint, oregano, thyme, turmeric, ginger, and cumin to bring the flavors together. Then use healthy oils to cook your meals and add healthy fats to your diet.

- **Meat**

  You may continue eating meat in moderation. Probably the biggest change you would have to make in your diet is to reduce your meat consumption. Do this gradually so that you won't feel like you're restricting yourself too much.

- **Nuts and seeds**

These healthy and tasty food items are satisfying and highly versatile. Options like almonds, chia seeds, flaxseeds, cashews, pistachios, and walnuts will make your diet more interesting whether you eat them for your snacks or add them to your dishes.

- **Plant-based proteins**

Even though you can eat meat while on the flexitarian diet, you can supplement your protein intake by including plant-based sources like tempeh, legumes, lentils, beans, and tofu.

- **Vegetables**

Veggies are the main focus of this diet. Vary your diet by adding different types of vegetables. Then make things more interesting for yourself by learning how to cook vegetables in different ways. Some examples of veggies to eat on this diet include leafy green veggies, peas, Brussels sprouts, bell peppers, green beans, corn, carrots, cauliflower, and sweet potato.

- **Whole grains**

These offer a lot of nutrients and fiber to add value to your diet. You can have whole grains like quinoa, brown rice, millet, amaranth, and even oatmeal at different times throughout the day.

Foods to Minimize

Part of the simple guidelines of this diet is to minimize a number of foods and food items. You don't have to eliminate these completely. Instead, you would just minimize your consumption of them so that you can focus on healthier options. The foods to minimize on the flexitarian diet are:

- **Added sweets and sugar** found in candy, cakes, soda, cookies, and donuts.
- **Fast food** like fries, milkshakes, burgers, and chicken nuggets.
- **Processed meat products** like bologna, sausage, and bacon.
- **Refined carbohydrates** like white rice, white bread, and assorted pastries.

Tips for Starting and Following the Flexitarian Diet

If you're new to the "diet scene" and you're looking for a diet that's easy but will improve your health, the flexitarian diet is the answer. As a flexitarian, you will basically be a vegetarian who still eats meat once in a while. The simplicity of this diet is its most attractive feature, and you can make things even easier for yourself by following these tips:

- **Come up with a strategy for starting the diet**

  First, learn everything you can about this diet. Unlike all the other diets, this step is a lot easier because there isn't much to learn about this diet aside from everything we covered here. After that, you can start coming up with a strategy for how to start and follow the diet. Then you can use the plan you create as a guide for when you actually start the diet.

- **Make small, healthy changes**

When it comes to starting this diet, you can decide how you will do it. But one of the best ways to approach the flexitarian diet is by making small, healthy changes to your diet. For instance, you can schedule a couple of meatless meals a week. Start with 1 to 2 meals each week and then move up from there.

As time goes by, you will be able to progress from the beginner to the advanced level and eventually become a flexitarian expert. As you will soon discover, this strategy will make it super easy for you to transition into the flexitarian diet. One day, you will just realize that you have already become a true flexitarian without even feeling like you tried too hard!

- **Come up with a routine**

Simple as this diet is, you still have to pay attention to the food you eat. While you make small changes to your diet, you should still try to make sure that you are eating balanced, healthy meals. To do this, you can come up with a routine for how to follow this simple eating pattern. You can even give meal planning a try. This is one of the easiest ways to create a routine around your diet.

- **Find healthier alternatives**

We have already established that going flexitarian doesn't mean that you have to say goodbye to certain foods or food groups. Even if you choose to focus more on plant-based foods, you still have the option to enjoy the food you eat by eating healthier alternatives to non-plant-based foods. For instance, instead of eating a burger with a beef patty, why don't you try one with a patty made of beans and beetroot. Since the flexitarian diet isn't very strict, making such changes is very easy.

- **Don't focus on restricting yourself**

If you want to succeed on the flexitarian diet, try not to focus on the part where you will gradually reduce your intake of meat and other "unhealthy" foods. Instead, try to focus on the positive changes you will be making on your diet. Since this diet is more plant-based, focus on finding healthy, tasty, and accessible food. Focus on increasing your intake of plants and when it's time for you to eat meat, think of it as a treat. Changing your perspective of how you will approach this diet makes it a more positive experience for you.

- **Experiment with plant-based food**

Since the flexitarian diet is primarily plant-based, you can make it more fun and sustainable by experimenting with different dishes. Go online and search for plant-based recipes, search for restaurants that offer vegan or vegetarian dishes, and you can even search for plant foods that you have never eaten in the past. Then give them a try.

Experimenting with plant-based foods will make things more interesting for you. As you discover different types of foods and dishes, you will also discover that plant-based foods aren't as "boring" as you might have thought in the first place. Eventually, you might even start choosing plant foods over meat or processed foods. When this happens, you can level up your flexitarian diet as you start moving towards healthier eating habits without even realizing it!

If you want to succeed on this diet, have fun with it! This is one of the easier diets and yet, it's still considered healthy and beneficial. After you have followed the flexitarian diet for some time, then you can determine whether you want to stick with it for the long-run or you would like to start following a more intense diet that has stricter rules and guidelines.

Chapter 6:
Intermittent Fasting

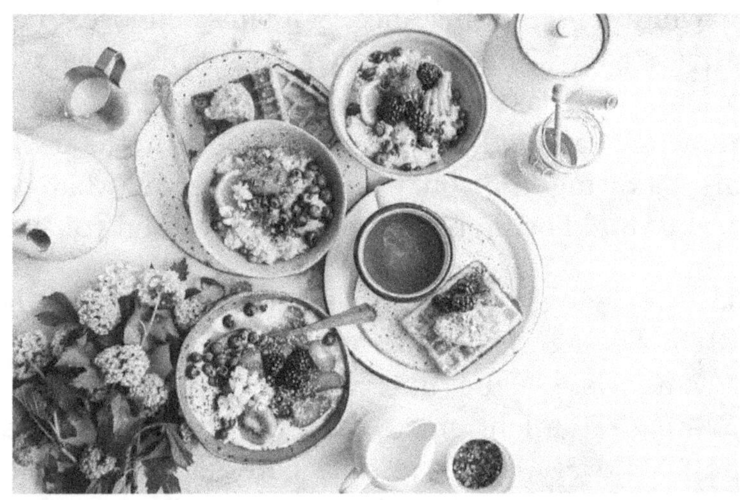

Fig. 7: Intermittent Fasting. Unsplash, by Brooke Lark, 2017, https://unsplash.com/photos/HlNcigvUi4Q/ Copyright 2017 by Brooke Lark/Unsplash.

Last but certainly not least in our list of super diets is intermittent fasting. This is another dietary trend that has taken the world by storm. Technically, though, intermittent fasting isn't a diet. It is more of an eating pattern since you will focus on the timings of your meals instead of the types of food you will be eating. All over the world, people are using intermittent fasting to improve their overall health, shed excess weight, and even make their lives simpler. Intermittent fasting is quite simple, and it can be followed in different ways. As you learn about this eating pattern in this final chapter, you can decide if it's the right super diet for you.

What Is Intermittent Fasting?

Intermittent fasting, or "IF" for short, is a type of eating pattern wherein you cycle between periods of fasting (also known as the fasting windows) and periods of eating (also known as the feasting windows). For instance, you may choose to fast for sixteen hours a day. This means that if your first meal would be at 8:00 a.m., your last meal should be at 4:00 p.m. After this time, you won't eat anything else until 8:00 a.m. the next day. If you start following IF, you wouldn't focus on what you eat. Instead, you would be more conscious about when you eat.

Just like the ketogenic diet, there are different methods of intermittent fasting. These methods vary in the length of the fasting windows. While intermittent fasting might seem overwhelming, it might make you feel better to know that everyone fasts every day. The time between the last meal you have each day (for instance, dinner is your last meal) and the first meal you have the next day (for instance, an early morning breakfast if your first meal) is time that you spend fasting. It's just that following IF makes you more aware of the time you spend fasting. In some cases, you would also lengthen this time to achieve your health goals faster.

Intermittent fasting is a customizable eating pattern as you can choose the IF method to follow. If this is your first time to try fasting, you can start with the simplest IF method to give your body time to adjust to fasting. Also, most people who start IF set their fasting window at night so that it includes the time when they sleep. This makes it easier for you to practice fasting as you won't feel hungry when you are sleeping. As time goes by, you can gradually increase your fasting window until you feel like you have reached your IF "sweet spot."

Another similarity between IF and the ketogenic diet is that both stimulate ketosis. During your fasting window, when your body runs out of glucose to burn for fuel, your body will enter the metabolic state known as ketosis where it starts burning fat for energy. This is one of the main reasons why a lot of people lose weight on this diet. But as soon as you have your first meal, your body goes back to its normal metabolic functions. So if you want to gain all of the benefits of IF, consistency is key.

Most Common Intermittent Fasting Methods

If you make the choice to follow IF, there are several methods you can follow. Choosing the method to follow depends on how experienced you are with fasting and what goals you want to achieve through intermittent fasting. As a beginner, it's recommended to choose the simplest method so as not to cause any adverse side effects. Here are the different IF methods to choose from:

5:2 Method

For this method, you will only fast for 2 days each week and then eat normally on the other 5 days. During your fasting days, you should only consume between 500 and 600 calories throughout the day. The 5:2 method is also known as the "Fast Diet." It's recommended to set your fasting days apart from each other with 1 to 2 days in between. This method can effectively help you lose weight if you follow it regularly. Also, you shouldn't try to eat more on your regular days to compensate for the calories you didn't consume on your fasting days.

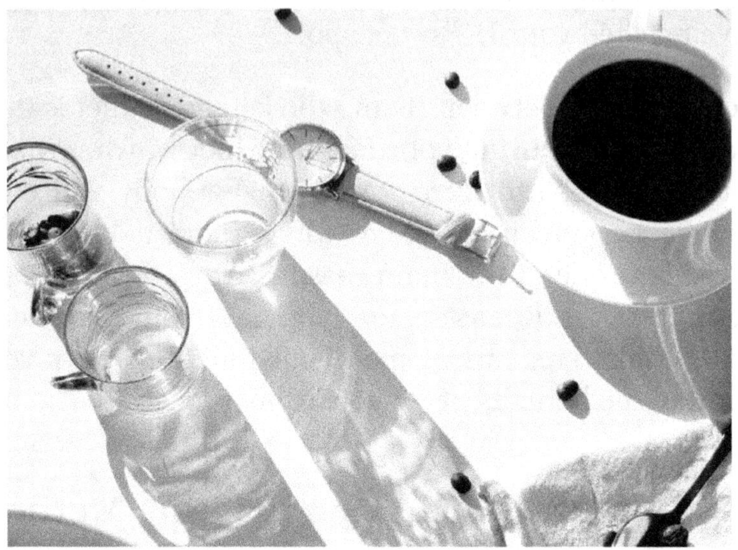

Fig. 8: IF Methods. Unsplash, by Jess Bailey, 2018, https://unsplash.com/photos/ULEUGITEbLs/ Copyright 2018 by Jess Bailey/Unsplash.

16/8 Method

For this method, you will follow IF every day wherein your fasting window will be 16 hours long and your feasting window will be 8 hours long. This is a flexible method as you can choose the times of your fasting and feasting windows. For instance, you can have your first meal at 10:00 a.m. and continue eating throughout the day until 6:00 p.m. From 6:01 p.m. to 9:59 a.m. (the next day), you will be fasting.

Such a schedule is quite easy to follow if you go to sleep regularly each night. But if you work at night and sleep in the morning, then you can flip this schedule to suit your lifestyle.

During your feasting window, just eat normally. If one of your goals is to lose weight, then you may gradually reduce your portions at each meal. Just make sure that you're still getting enough nutrients throughout the day so you don't end up getting sick.

As a beginner, fasting for 16 hours straight might be too much for you. In such a case, you can increase your feasting window to 10 hours and reduce your fasting window down to 14 hours. After a few weeks when you feel like your body has adjusted to IF, then you can start following the 16/8 method.

Alternate-Day Fasting

For this method, your fasting days would occur every other day. Although this is one of the more common IF methods, it has its own variations. For instance, during your alternate fasting days, you don't have to fast completely. Instead, you would simply reduce your caloric intake to just 500 calories. As a beginner, this can be a good option for you. If you choose to start with alternate-day fasting, you shouldn't dive into full fasts right away. Instead, you should ease into the eating pattern to give your body (and mind) time to adjust.

Warrior Diet

This is probably the most extreme IF method, which means that it's not recommended for beginners. The simpler version of this method involves consuming minimal amounts of raw veggies and fruits throughout the day and then having a huge meal for dinner. The more extreme version of this diet involves not eating anything throughout the day and only giving yourself up to 4 hours at the end of the day to eat one huge meal. And you would be doing this every day.

If you haven't tried fasting in the past, you might not want to opt for this method right away as it could cause a lot of unpleasant experiences for you. But if you do try to follow this method sometime in the future, you should learn how to follow it properly. That way, you don't risk experiencing adverse side effects that will compromise your health and safety.

Spontaneous Meal Skipping

Although this isn't considered a "real" method of IF, you can use it to practice before you start with the other IF methods. Here, you will simply skip meals from time to time if you don't have time to eat, you just don't feel like eating, or you don't feel hungry during your regular mealtimes. Spontaneous meal skipping allows you to experience the feeling of fasting without having to stick with a rigorous schedule yet. When you feel like you can already handle regular fasting, then you can choose your own IF method.

The Benefits of the Mediterranean Diet

Intermittent fasting has become hugely popular for a number of reasons. This eating pattern offers several benefits both in terms of health and lifestyle. As you consider if this can be your next big life choice, these are the potential benefits you can look forward to:

Simplicity

If you are looking for a dietary change that can simplify your life, IF fits the bill. Since you will be shortening the time when you will eat your meals, you don't have to plan what you will eat from morning until night and everything in between. The shorter your feasting window is, the simpler your life becomes. Think about it: If you follow the warrior method, you only have to plan one complete meal each day. For the rest of the day, you simply have to drink water, plain tea, coffee, or broth if you're feeling hungry. As you start out, you may have to plan and prepare for IF, but once you get the hang of it, your life will become a lot simpler.

Apart from being simple, IF is much easier than following a strict diet. You don't have to eliminate any types of food from your diet while following IF. Of course, it's still recommended to consume whole, natural foods to ensure that you will always stay at the peak of health. But for this eating pattern, you don't have to restrict yourself in terms of what you should eat.

Weight Loss

One of the most common benefits of IF is weight loss. During your fasting periods, your body will achieve ketosis, the metabolic state that turns your body into a fat-burning machine. If you can maintain consistency and even lengthen the duration of your fasts, then you will soon shed those stubborn excess pounds. Even if you don't reduce your portions, you can still potentially lose weight. Since your feasting windows each day have been reduced, you won't be eating as many meals throughout the day as you used to.

Cognitive Health

Intermittent fasting can also improve your memory, thinking, and other cognitive skills. The reason for this is that ketones—the fuel molecules produced during ketosis—are a more efficient source of fuel for the brain. This means that during your fasting windows, your brain may actually become healthier and more powerful as it runs on fuel generated from burning your body's fat stores.

Heart Health

Another major organ that can benefit from IF is your heart. As you follow this eating pattern, you may experience improvements in your resting heart rate and blood pressure. This is an amazing benefit since a healthy heart can help maintain your overall health too.

Disease Prevention

By following IF, you can lower your risk of developing other diseases too. For one, you can avoid obesity through IF. Since this diet promotes weight loss, you don't have to worry about gaining excess weight while on it. In fact, if you already suffer from obesity, you can lose the excess weight you have always been trying to get rid of.

As your heart health improves and you avoid obesity too, this helps reduce your risk of developing diabetes, another chronic disease that can make your life very difficult. Intermittent fasting even has the potential to prevent some forms of cancer. For those who are undergoing chemotherapy, fasting before each treatment session can help improve their recovery and reduce mortality rates.

Improved Longevity

With all the benefits you can look forward to by following IF, you can also expect to live a longer, healthier life. Think about it: If you don't get sick, you maintain a healthy weight, and you don't experience high levels of stress because your life is simpler, longevity is a natural consequence.

If you want to enjoy all of these wonderful benefits, you must learn how to follow intermittent fasting correctly. Simple as it is, there is a right way to do IF and a wrong way to do it. The right way leads to benefits while the wrong way can potentially lead to a number of risks and adverse side effects. And when you have gotten used to this eating pattern, you can even combine it with a diet such as keto to get even more benefits!

Potential Risks and Side Effects

Although intermittent fasting is a healthy super diet—or eating pattern—it's not necessarily recommended for everyone. There are certain people who should think twice before following this diet, especially since it can get quite intense. If you belong to any of these groups, you may want to re-consider going on IF:

- You suffer from or have a history of eating disorders.
- You are underweight.
- You have low blood sugar.
- You suffer from type 1 diabetes or you have issues with your blood sugar levels.

- You are taking medications to treat or manage a certain disease.
- You are pregnant or breastfeeding.
- In some cases, IF isn't recommended for women because it changes the internal workings of the body.

If you fall under any of these groups but you still want to follow IF, speak with your doctor first before doing so. Your doctor can tell you whether this eating pattern is safe for you or not. If your doctor gives you the green light, you can come up with a plan for which method to follow and how to approach intermittent fasting.

Even if you are at the peak of your health, there are still some risks and side effects you should look out for if you choose to fast intermittently. By knowing these side effects, you can prepare yourself for them and even take the necessary steps to avoid them:

- **Feeling "hangry"**

  The word "hangry" means feeling angry because of your hunger. If this is your first time to try fasting, this is something that you might experience frequently. Although you won't feel the negative effects of your "hanger," it might take a toll on your relationships. For instance, if you are a stay-at-home-mom and you always get angry at your kids because you're hungry, this might cause a rift in your relationship. This is why you shouldn't try the extreme methods of IF right away as you might end up alienating everyone around you.

- **Other mood changes**

Aside from feeling hangry, you might experience other extreme changes in your mood too, especially in the beginning. You may feel anxious, grouchy, or even discouraged. Probably the best thing you can do to avoid this is to find things to distract yourself with. If you are always busy with something, you won't keep focusing on your hunger and on the fact that your next feasting window is hours away.

- **Developing an obsession with food**

Restricting yourself too much by setting very long fasting periods might result in developing an obsession with food. For instance, throughout your fasting window, all you can think about is what you will eat, how many hours are left before your feasting window, how much you will eat, and anything else related to food. If you notice that you can think of nothing else but food while you are fasting, then you may have to change your strategy.

- **Brain fog and fatigue**

These effects are very common, especially in the beginning of your IF journey. As your body adjusts to this eating pattern, you may experience times when you just can't think clearly (brain fog) or you are too tired to function (fatigue). The key here is to consume healthy, whole foods to give you enough energy to last throughout your fasting windows.

- **Low levels of blood sugar**

If you experience dizziness, headaches, or nausea that doesn't go away, these can be indications that your levels of blood sugar have dropped too low. This is why those who suffer from type 1 diabetes shouldn't follow IF. If you end up becoming hypoglycemic because of fasting too much or for too long, this can be very harmful to your health.

- **Constipation**

You might experience this side effect if you're not getting enough fiber, protein, vitamins, and fluid from your diet. Even if you only eat a single meal throughout the day, you must make sure that the meal you eat counts. Focus on healthy, nutrient-rich foods so you don't end up experiencing constipation and other bowel issues.

- **Hair loss**

Surprising as this might seem, you can even lose your hair as a consequence of going too extreme with your intermittent fasting efforts. Hair loss might happen if you don't get enough nutrients from the foods you eat. In particular, if you don't get enough B vitamins and protein, this might be something you will go through.

- **Sleep disturbances**

While you can enjoy better sleep while on IF, the beginning of your journey might be plagued with sleep disturbances. Probably the most common cause of this is feeling hungry. As your body adjusts to fasting, strong feelings of hunger might keep you awake at night.

- **For women, menstrual cycle changes**

  This is one of the reasons why intermittent fasting isn't always recommended for women. If you lose a lot of weight and you aren't getting enough nutrients all the time, you might notice changes in your menstrual cycle. In some cases, your periods might even stop completely. In such a case, you should stop fasting or at least change the IF method you're following.

As you can see, intermittent fasting isn't risk-free. This is why you should learn more about it, especially about the method you plan to follow. That way, you can make sure that you will follow the method correctly to ensure the improvement of your health and well-being.

Foods to Eat and Avoid

Since intermittent fasting is an eating pattern, you don't have to focus too much on the foods you eat. Of course, if you want to improve your health, you should still focus on healthy foods while following IF. Let's take a look at the most recommended foods to eat and the food items you should try to avoid to enjoy all of the benefits of this super diet.

Foods to Eat

Whole, natural, healthy foods are your best bet if you want to get all of the nutrients your body needs even if you are fasting. If you want to make meal plans for your intermittent fasting schedule, here are some of the best options to include:

- **Beverages and liquids** like broth, plain coffee, plain tea, red wine (on occasion), and water.
- **Dairy products** like fortified milk, plain yogurt, and cheese.
- **Fatty fish** like mackerel, salmon, sardines, tuna, and trout.
- **Fruits** like apples, apricots, blueberries, blackberries, cherries, papaya, peaches, pears, plums, raspberries, oranges, and watermelon.
- **Lean proteins** like fish, Greek yogurt, lean meat, seafood, tofu, and whitefish.
- **Legumes** like chickpeas, lentils, and peanuts.
- **Minimally-processed grains** like whole-grain bagels, bread, and crackers.
- **Nuts** like almonds, Brazil nuts, cashews, hazelnuts, macadamia nuts, pecans, pistachios, and walnuts.
- **Smoothies** made from fresh fruits, veggies, and other healthy ingredients.
- **Vegetables** like arugula, cabbage, chard, collard greens, kale, potatoes, and spinach.

Foods to Avoid

While you can technically eat anything that you want while on IF, there are still certain foods you may want to avoid, especially since you are working to improve your health. To ensure your health while following IF, here are some foods to stay away from:

- Alcoholic beverages like beer and cocktails.
- Processed meat products like bacon, hot dogs, salami, and bologna.

- Processed savory snacks like microwave popcorn and snack chips.
- Refined grains like pasta, pizza dough, white bread, white flour, and white rice.
- Sauces and condiments with added sugar like ketchup and barbecue sauce.
- Sugary beverages like fruit juices and sodas.
- Sugary foods like cakes, candies, cereals, cookies, and granola bars.
- Trans fats like those in baked goods, fried foods, non-dairy coffee creamer, refrigerated dough, shortening, and stick margarine.

During your fasting periods, you shouldn't eat any solid foods. In the beginning, if you feel really hungry, you can have a light and healthy snack like a handful of nuts or a couple of fresh vegetable sticks. Otherwise, you can ease your hunger by drinking a lot of water and zero-calorie drinks like plain tea and coffee. You may also drink broth for a filling snack while fasting.

Tips for Starting and Following Intermittent Fasting

Intermittent fasting doesn't have to be complicated. Now that you know the basics of this eating pattern, you should have a better understanding of what it entails. Although you should learn more about the IF method you will choose, there are some general guidelines you can follow to make your IF journey smoother and easier:

- **Identify your health goals**

  Before anything else, you must think about your health goals. Whether you plan to follow IF or any other super diet, you must first know your reasons for wanting to change your eating habits. If you can identify your health goals, creating a plan for your IF journey becomes simpler. For instance, if you want to lose weight, you can choose a method that will help you achieve this. Writing down your health goals gives you a guide for how you will approach this eating pattern.

- **Think about the IF method you will choose**

After identifying your goals, the next thing to think about is the IF method to follow. We have already gone through the most common methods you can choose from. Now all you have to do is to decide which one to start with. The great thing about IF is that you can choose a method and use it as a guide. Then you can customize the method you have chosen so that it suits your own needs, preferences, and lifestyle.

- **Keep yourself busy**

This is one of the most useful tips to overcome the challenges of IF. Expect to feel hungry all the time, especially in the beginning. Of course, if you aren't doing anything, you will only focus on your hunger. You might even develop an obsession with food. To avoid this, find ways to distract yourself and be more productive. If you go to work every day, this is much easier. But if you are normally at home, then you have to think of creative ways to focus on other things. Before you know it, your feasting window will arrive where you can enjoy a healthy, well-deserved meal.

- **Make sure you're well-hydrated**

Whether you are in your fasting window or feasting window, you should always make sure that you are well-hydrated. For this, water is your best option. But you can also opt for non-caloric beverages, especially during your fasting windows. When it's time for your feasting windows, you can opt for more indulgent beverages. The key is to make sure that you are drinking enough liquids throughout the day. Dehydration can be very dangerous so you should avoid it at all costs.

- **Make your calories count**

When you start fasting intermittently, you don't have to reduce your portions right away. Remember that reducing your eating hours will automatically result in a reduction of your caloric intake too. Instead of focusing on reducing your caloric intake, make sure that all the calories you eat throughout the day count. Even if you are fasting, you must still aim to consume all of the daily recommended vitamins, minerals, and nutrients each day. This is especially important as you start following more extreme methods like the warrior diet. If you don't want to develop deficiencies or experience any of the potential side effects of IF, make sure you're not restricting yourself too much.

- **Avoid binging or overeating**

Just as you shouldn't restrict yourself during your feasting windows, you should also avoid binging or overeating when your fasting windows end. This is a very common issue that a lot of beginners at IF experience. Because of the hunger you feel after fasting, you might end up consuming more than the recommended calories each day. If you do this, don't expect to experience the potential benefits of IF, especially weight loss. When it's time for you to start eating again, stick with your normal portions and eating habits. You don't have to compensate for the meals or snacks you missed while fasting.

- **Learn how to listen to your body**

This particular tip will be very useful to you whether you follow IF or any of the super diets we have already discussed. Your success on IF lies in your ability to listen to your body and observe the changes that happen each day. By tuning in to your body and being more aware, you will know whether intermittent fasting is improving your health or if you are starting to experience the negative side effects. As you observe these things, you can either stick with the method you have chosen because it is working for you or you can choose another method that will help you reach your health goals.

- **Allow yourself some flexibility**

If you experience some setbacks, especially in the beginning, that's okay. Be flexible with yourself and with the IF method you have chosen. For instance, if you have decided on the 5:2 method but on your first fasting day, you feel too hungry to function, allow yourself to eat a light snack. Don't allow yourself to feel restricted, frustrated, or even depressed because of this eating pattern, otherwise, you might give up on it too soon.

- **Break your fast properly**

Finally, you should learn how to enter into your feasting window properly. For one, you shouldn't gorge on a full-course meal as soon as your fasting window ends. Eating too much after fasting for hours will give you stomach pains. Hungry as you are, it's better to opt for a light yet satisfying meal at the beginning of your feasting window. If you come up with a plan for how to go about your fasting and feasting windows, you may want to include the first meals you will eat after each time you fast. That way, you won't reach for the first thing you see, which usually tends to be something unhealthy.

Chapter 7:
Choosing the Best Diet for Your Health

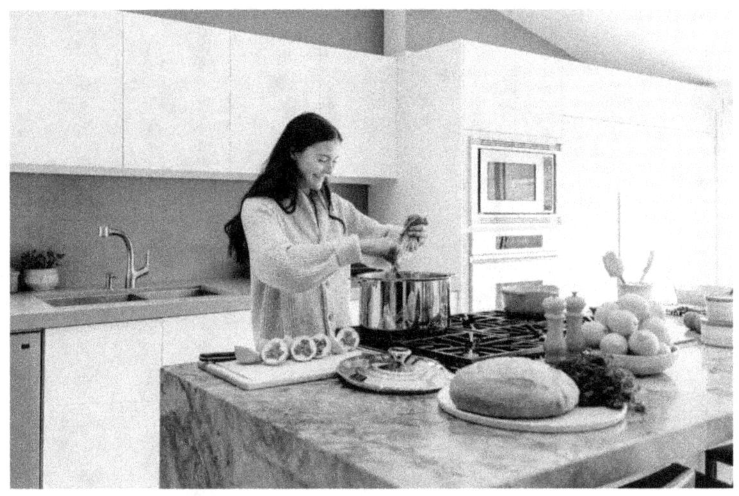

Fig. 9: Choosing Your Diet. Unsplash, by Jason Briscoe, 2019, https://unsplash.com/photos/GrdJp16CPk8/ Copyright 2019 by Jason Briscoe/Unsplash.

There you have it—the super diets that will change your life. No matter how bad your current eating habits are, you can clean up your life and improve your health by choosing any one of these diets. As you have learned, some diets are simpler and easier than others. There are also diets that will give you faster results. Ultimately, you will enjoy the potential benefits of these diets if you know how to follow them correctly and you maintain consistency.

Now that you have learned the basics of these super diets, what more is there for you to discover? In this chapter, you will learn how to choose the best diet for your own lifestyle. Choosing the right diet requires thought, planning, and self-reflection. You must know what you want, what you need, and what you are aiming to achieve. By knowing all of these things, you will surely find a diet that will make things better for you health-wise. If you really want to know how to make the best decision in terms of choosing a new diet, you must first consider a number of factors.

Factors to Consider

Knowing all about the healthiest super diets is just one step in finding the perfect diet to suit your lifestyle. By learning the basics of each diet, you will have a better idea of which diet you would like to choose. But before making that final choice, consider the following factors:

- **Your health and fitness goals**

  People who start new diets always have a reason for doing so. The most common reasons include weight loss, the management or treatment of a medical condition, or to improve their health. Before considering which super diet to follow, think about your own health and fitness goals. Make a list of everything you want to achieve through the diet. This will help narrow down your options and make it easier for you to decide.

- **Your current state of health**

After you have written down your goals, it's time to examine your current state of health. If you are at the peak of health right now, you may choose any of the super diets you've learned about. But if you suffer from any kind of medical condition or you have a high risk of developing one, then you have to choose your diet carefully. Go back to the potential risks and side effects of each diet before making a choice. Also, it would be best to consult with your doctor first to help you decide.

- **Your lifestyle**

It would be very difficult to dive into the vegan diet if you are a heavy meat eater who isn't used to plant-based foods. Although you would like to improve your health by making this change, choosing a diet that's too far from your current diet and lifestyle would be very challenging. Instead, you can opt for a diet that is somewhat similar to your current one. Start with that, and then gradually transition into the diet you want to follow long-term.

It would also be useful to consider your home life. If everyone in your family is following a certain diet and you want to follow one that's drastically different, you would have to put in a lot of effort to do so. If you think that you can pull it off, go ahead! If not, you may want to opt for a diet that will still help you reach your goals but will also fit into your lifestyle.

- **Your activity levels**

Generally, diets work better when you pair them with regular exercise. However, if you will opt for one of the more extreme diets (for instance, the warrior method of IF), you might have to adjust your workout routines. You have two choices here. You can either match your diet to your workout routines or you can adjust your workout routines to the diet you will choose. The key here is to make sure that you are getting enough exercise each day while getting enough nourishment to fuel your workouts.

- **The rules and guidelines of the diet**

As you consider which diet to choose, think about whether you want one that offers a lot of flexibility or a structured diet that has specific rules you should follow. If you feel more motivated when you have a set of rules and guidelines to follow, then you may choose a diet that offers such—like the ketogenic diet. But if you don't want to feel like you have to follow rigid rules when making changes to your diet, you can opt for a more flexible type of diet—like the flexitarian diet. Think about what motivates you and how well you follow rules. This is another important determining factor that will help you make the best decision.

- **The sustainability of the diet**

Finally, think about the sustainability of the diet or how realistic it is for you. If you want to enjoy the many benefits these diets have to offer, you must follow the one you choose for a long time. In fact, making it part of your lifestyle would be ideal. That is unless your doctor only recommends that you follow one of these diets for a certain period of time to help with the treatment of some medical condition. Otherwise, it's better to choose a sustainable diet.

When thinking about which diet to start with, ask yourself, "Will I be able to follow this diet for the rest of my life?" If the answer to this question is, "no" or if you keep coming up with excuses for not going through with it, move on. But if the diet makes you feel excited and you feel like you can easily incorporate it into your life now, go for it!

As you consider all of these factors in your decision-making process, you will discover that choosing the right diet isn't that difficult. But one thing that you may have noticed is that the super diets have a lot of things in common. These are:

- They encourage you to reflect on your current diet, eating habits, and health.
- They encourage you to learn how to be more aware of your body so that you can listen to it as you make gradual changes in your diet.
- They encourage you to focus on whole, natural, nutrient-dense foods while gradually eliminating junk and processed foods from your diet.
- They encourage you to make changes and modifications in your diet as needed even though you would choose one of them as your basis.

All of these are amazing health habits that you will learn as you decide to follow one of these super diets. These basic habits will prepare you for a long-term journey of health and happiness.

After you have chosen a diet by considering all of these factors and everything you have learned about the individual diets, you can gradually incorporate the diet into your life. As you do this, try to reassess the changes you are making. Do this regularly. For this, you need to listen to your body and be aware of the changes you are making. For instance, you have chosen to follow IF and you have started with the 14/10 method (an easier variation of the 16/8 method).

After a few weeks of following this method, try to see how you feel about it. Are you able to follow it easily or are you still struggling with the length of the fasting window? If you feel like you have already adjusted to the diet, you can level up and try the 16/8 method. But if you feel like you're still struggling with it, then you can stick with the current method for a few more weeks. Finding and choosing a diet isn't a one-time thing. It's a journey that you will have to go on to achieve your health and fitness goals.

Does the "Perfect Diet" Exist?

No, it doesn't.

There is no such thing as a "perfect diet," but there are diets that can potentially suit your life perfectly. Educating yourself is an important part of the process of choosing the right diet. Fortunately, you have already done that! At this point, you should already have a good idea of which diet is the right one. You already know what the super diets are and how to start them, and you already know the factors to consider to help you choose.

Everything you have learned here will enable you to narrow down your options until you have zoned into the diet that will change your life. No matter what your health goals are, any one of these diets can potentially improve your overall health and well-being. Just make sure that you follow through with the diet you have chosen, especially if you want to enjoy all of the benefits it has to offer. Also, keep the following tips and considerations in mind:

- Pair your diet with regular exercise or an active lifestyle.
- Vary the foods you eat to keep you motivated.
- Consult with your doctor if you experience any adverse side effects after a few days or weeks of following the diet.
- Try to start your diet with a positive mindset instead of forcing yourself to change your eating habits.
- Allow yourself to make mistakes, then keep going.
- Come up with a backup plan for when you discover that the diet you have chosen isn't working for you.
- Always drink a lot of water no matter which diet you have chosen.

As you prepare to start your diet, take a moment to sit down, prepare, and come up with a plan. As you are doing this, try to find ways to inspire and motivate yourself too. For instance, you can join forums or online communities for the diet you have chosen. Such groups give you a place to talk about your experiences and learn how other people have overcome the challenges of your chosen diet. If you want to find the perfect diet, you need to put in the effort. And when you have settled into the diet of your choice, you may realize that it is indeed the perfect diet for you.

Customizing Your Diet to Suit Your Needs

After choosing a diet to follow, you can either follow it or make it easier for you to follow by making a couple of modifications to it. To do this, you must first understand how the diet works and what its basic rules are. All diets have their own rules, even the simplest ones. And these rules exist for a reason. Without rules, you won't know where to start or what you need to do to achieve the benefits you are aiming for.

Of course, you don't always have to follow rules strictly no matter what diet you choose to follow. If you really want to follow a certain diet but you feel like some of the rules are too restrictive, then you can customize your diet to make it easier for you. Customizing your diet doesn't mean that you will drastically change the rules. It just means that you will make some changes to the things that you feel don't work for you while still following the basic principles of the diet. To help you out, here are some ways to customize the diet you have chosen:

- **Speak with a nutritionist or a registered dietitian**

  Before you start making any changes to your diet, you may want to have a conversation with experts first. Speak with a nutritionist or a registered dietitian about the diet you want to follow and the possible changes you want to make. That way, you can still make sure that you're following a healthy diet even though you won't follow the rules strictly.

- **Make a list of your favorite foods and try to see if you can include these in your diet**

  This is a great way to motivate yourself to follow the diet you have chosen. No matter how restrictive your diet is, you can still enjoy your favorite foods. After making a list of your favorite foods, go through the list of recommended foods of the diet you have chosen. Check all of the foods that you can still continue eating. For your favorite foods that you would have to avoid, try to find healthier alternatives for them that won't break the rules of your diet.

- **Make changes as you go along**

  When it comes to customizing your diet, you don't have to do it right away. As you follow the diet, you will discover what works, what doesn't, and what improvements you can make. As you discover these things, jot them down on a journal or notebook. Every two weeks or so, go through your notes and make changes as needed. Keep doing this until you don't find anything else that you want or need to change in your diet.

The most important thing about diets that you should remember is that there is no one-size-fits-all diet. Even if some diets might work for a lot of people, they might not work for you. If you reach a point where you don't think you can continue with the diet no matter how hard you have tried, you should consider throwing in the towel. Then you can choose another super diet. Hopefully, one that will be more sustainable for you.

<u>Conclusion:</u>
Which Super Diet Is Right for You?

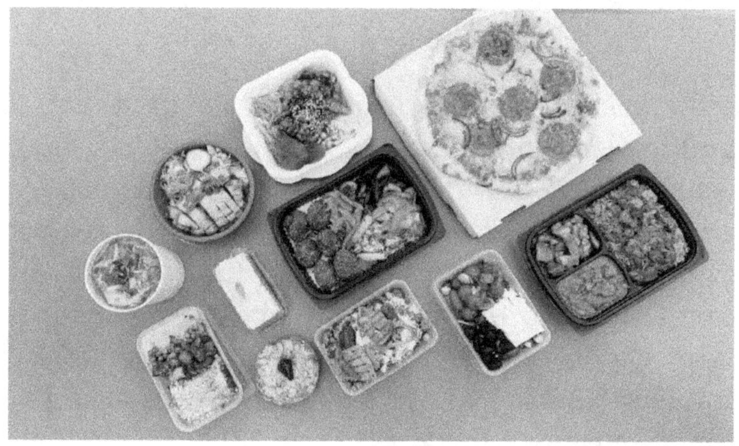

Fig. 10: Different Diets. Unsplash, by Cristiano Pinto, 2020, https://unsplash.com/photos/2lWGQ02DGL8/ Copyright 2020 by Cristiano Pinto/Unsplash.

Mediterranean? Keto? Vegan? Paleo? Flexitarian? Intermittent Fasting?

Which super diet is the right one for you?

Now that you have learned all of the fundamentals of these incredibly healthy diets, you can make the best decision as to which one you will incorporate into your life. As you have learned throughout this book, all of these diets offer something unique that will change your life for the better.

If you have made the choice to start some kind of diet, it means that you already have some health and fitness goals in mind. To choose the best super diet for yourself, you may want to write these goals down and use them to guide you. From the beginning of this book all the way to the end, you discovered the healthiest and most beneficial super diets out there. For each diet, we talked about what the diets were all about, what benefits you can expect from them, and even the potential risks and downsides to look forward to.

Beyond the basics, you also learned the foods to eat, foods to avoid, and foods to minimize as you follow these diets. Then we ended each chapter with a number of practical tips and strategies for you to start following the diets and stick with them long-term. But your learning journey didn't end there. In the last chapter, we also discussed the factors you must consider before you choose a diet to start with. This chapter is very important as it enables you to make the best decision based on the factors discussed.

This eBook has delivered exactly what it promised—a complete list of all the best super diets out there along with enough information to help you understand what makes them so awesome. Now that you have learned the basics, it's time for you to dig deeper after you have chosen the diet that would suit your own lifestyle. Your health is one of your greatest treasures. If you want to take care of it, you must make positive changes in your life. Whether you want to lose weight, improve your health, or just want to get with the trends, you can't go wrong by picking any of these diets.

There is no time like the present to change your life for the better. Challenging as it might be to change your diet and eating habits, these changes will cause a ripple effect as they improve the different aspects of your life. By now, you should already have a good idea of which diet (or diets) are ideal for your own situation. The next step is to continue learning about the diet you have chosen. Then you should come up with a plan for how to follow it.

Don't forget to include the tips and strategies you learned here. Once you have your plan, you can start easing into the diet of your choice. As you do, continue to listen to your body so that you can determine whether the diet is working for you or against you. Good luck with the diet you have chosen and always remember to give yourself a break once in a while. You've got this!

References

4 Paleo Tips to Escape Common Beginner Traps. (2017, May 8). Paleo Leap. https://paleoleap.com/4-paleo-tips-escape-common-beginner-traps/

Bradford, A. (2015, November 18). *Mediterranean Diet: Foods, Benefits & Risks*. Live Science. https://www.livescience.com/52832-mediterranean-diet.html

Bradley, S. (2019, November 11). *10 Intermittent Fasting Side Effects That Might Mean It's Not A Great Fit For You*. Women's Health. https://www.womenshealthmag.com/weight-loss/a29657614/intermittent-fasting-side-effects/

Brazier, Y. (2020, January 17). *Mediterranean Diet: Facts, Benefits, and Tips*. Medical News Today. https://www.medicalnewstoday.com/articles/149090

Carroll, C. (2020, April 23). *What Is the Flexitarian Diet?* Verywell Fit. https://www.verywellfit.com/how-flexitarian-diet-works-4588694

Castaneda, R. (2020). *Intermittent Fasting: Foods to Eat and Avoid*. US News & World Report. https://health.usnews.com/wellness/food/articles/intermittent-fasting-foods-to-eat-and-avoid

Clarke, C. (2018a, April 7). *The 10 Best Tips for Keto Diet Success*. Ruled Me. https://www.ruled.me/the-10-best-tips-for-keto-diet-success/

Clarke, C. (2018b, July 21). *How to Start a Keto Diet: 3 Simple Steps to Keto Success.* Ruled Me. https://www.ruled.me/how-to-start-a-keto-diet/

Clear, J. (2012, December 10). *The Beginner's Guide to Intermittent Fasting.* James Clear. https://jamesclear.com/the-beginners-guide-to-intermittent-fasting

Cording, J. (2019, August 28). *Is the Secret to Losing Weight More About When You Eat Than What?* Shape. https://www.shape.com/healthy-eating/diet-tips/potential-intermittent-fasting-benefits-not-worth-dieting-risks

Disadvantages of Mediterranean Diet. (n.d.). India Parenting. Retrieved September 10, 2020, from https://www.indiaparenting.com/disadvantages-of-mediterranean-diet.html

Eenfeldt, A. (2019, February 21). *Diet Doctor.* Diet Doctor. https://www.dietdoctor.com/low-carb/keto

Fletcher, J. (2019, April 5). *Intermittent fasting for weight loss: 5 tips to start.* Medical News Today. https://www.medicalnewstoday.com/articles/324882

Food52. (2016, January 18). *10 Must-Read Tips If You're Thinking About Going Vegan.* SELF. https://www.self.com/story/must-read-tips-going-vegan

Forrest, C. (2019, October 2). *Eight Vegan Diet Dangers (One Is Irreversible).* Clean Eating Kitchen. https://www.cleaneatingkitchen.com/vegan-diet-dangers-health/

Frey, M. (2020, March 13). *How to Make Your Own Rules for Weight Loss*. Verywell Fit. https://www.verywellfit.com/how-to-follow-a-make-your-own-rules-diet-4153881

Fung, J. (2019, April 25). *Diet Doctor*. Diet Doctor. https://www.dietdoctor.com/intermittent-fasting

Girdwain, J., & Walsh, K. (2019, March 28). *The Paleo Diet for Beginners*. Shape. https://www.shape.com/healthy-eating/diet-tips/beginners-guide-paleo-diet

Gunnars, K. (2018a, July 24). *Mediterranean Diet 101: A Meal Plan and Beginner's Guide*. Healthline. https://www.healthline.com/nutrition/mediterranean-diet-meal-plan

Gunnars, K. (2018b, August 1). *The Paleo Diet — A Beginner's Guide + Meal Plan*. Healthline. https://www.healthline.com/nutrition/paleo-diet-meal-plan-and-menu

Gunnars, K. (2020a, January 1). *6 Popular Ways to Do Intermittent Fasting*. Healthline. https://www.healthline.com/nutrition/6-ways-to-do-intermittent-fasting

Gunnars, K. (2020b, April 20). *Intermittent Fasting 101 — The Ultimate Beginner's Guide*. Healthline. https://www.healthline.com/nutrition/intermittent-fasting-guide

Hackett, J. (2020, January 31). *What Is Veganism?* The Spruce Eats. https://www.thespruceeats.com/what-do-vegans-eat-3376824

Helms, N. (2019, June 20). *Ketogenic diet: What are the risks?* UChicago Medicine. https://www.uchicagomedicine.org/forefront/health-and-wellness-articles/ketogenic-diet-what-are-the-risks

Hendricks, S. (2019, January 18). *7 Foods You Should Avoid on the Mediterranean Diet.* Insider. https://www.insider.com/mediterranean-diet-foods-not-to-eat-2019-1

Huggins Salomon, S. (2019). *8 Scientific Health Benefits of the Mediterranean Diet.* Everyday Health. https://www.everydayhealth.com/mediterranean-diet/scientific-health-benefits-mediterranean-diet/

Intermittent Fasting: What is it, and how does it work? (n.d.). Johns Hopkins Medicine. https://www.hopkinsmedicine.org/health/wellness-and-prevention/intermittent-fasting-what-is-it-and-how-does-it-work

Jhaveri, A. (2017, December 11). *A Beginner's Guide to Going Vegan and Living Your Best Plant-Based Life.* Greatist. https://greatist.com/eat/what-is-a-vegan-diet

Jitchotvisut, J. (2019, April 25). *5 Potential Drawbacks of Following a Vegan Diet.* Insider. https://www.insider.com/the-potential-risks-of-being-vegan-2019-4

Kamb, S. (2020, May 26). *Intermittent Fasting For Beginners: Should You Skip Breakfast?* Nerd Fitness. https://www.nerdfitness.com/blog/a-beginners-guide-to-intermittent-fasting/#tips_for_intermittent_fasting

Karadsheh, S. (2019, May 1). *What is the Mediterranean Diet and How to Follow It*. The Mediterranean Dish. https://www.themediterraneandish.com/7-ways-follow-mediterranean-diet/

Keto Diet Plan for Beginners. (n.d.). Atkins. Retrieved September 10, 2020, from https://www.atkins.com/how-it-works/library/articles/how-to-start-a-keto-diet-7-tips-for-beginners

Krampf, M. (2020, January 15). *15 Best Keto Diet Tips & Tricks For Beginners*. Wholesome Yum. https://www.wholesomeyum.com/keto-diet-tips-for-beginners/

Laurence, E. (2019, April 4). *9 Mediterranean Diet Benefits That Explain Why Experts Love It So Much*. Well+Good. https://www.wellandgood.com/mediterranean-diet-benefits/

Lawler, M. (2019, April 22). *What Are the Benefits and Risks of the Paleo Diet?* Everyday Health. https://www.everydayhealth.com/diet-nutrition/paleo-diet/what-are-risks-benefits-paleo-diet/

Lee, S. (2014, February 25). *How To Choose Your Best Diet*. Body Building. https://www.bodybuilding.com/fun/how-to-choose-the-best-diet-for-you.html

Mawer, R. (2018). *The Ketogenic Diet: A Detailed Beginner's Guide to Keto*. Healthline. https://www.healthline.com/nutrition/ketogenic-diet-101

Mayo Clinic Staff. (2017). *Paleo diet: What is it and Why is it So Popular?* Mayo Clinic. https://www.mayoclinic.org/healthy-lifestyle/nutrition-and-healthy-eating/in-depth/paleo-diet/art-20111182

Mediterranean Diet. (2018). US News. https://health.usnews.com/best-diet/mediterranean-diet

Mercy Health. (2018, April 27). *What is the Ketogenic Diet? Learn the Potential Benefits and Risks.* Mercy Health Blog. https://blog.mercy.com/ketogenic-diet-risks-benefits/

Migala, J. (2019a, January 3). *What Is the Mediterranean Diet? Your Ultimate Guide to the Heart-Healthy Eating Philosophy.* Everyday Health. https://www.everydayhealth.com/mediterranean-diet/guide/

Migala, J. (2019b, August 23). *What Are the Benefits and Risks of the Keto Diet?* Everyday Health. https://www.everydayhealth.com/diet-nutrition/ketogenic-diet/what-are-benefits-risks-keto-diet/

Migala, J. (2019c, December 18). *8 Ways to Follow the Mediterranean Diet for Better Health.* Eating Well. http://www.eatingwell.com/article/16372/8-ways-to-follow-the-mediterranean-diet-for-better-health/

Miller, K., & Mahtani, N. (2018, March 15). *What Is The Keto Diet, Exactly?* Women's Health. https://www.womenshealthmag.com/weight-loss/a19434332/what-is-the-keto-diet/

Orenstein, B. W. (2019, June 27). *Paleo Diet 101: Beginner's Guide of What to Eat and How It Works.* Everyday Health. https://www.everydayhealth.com/diet-nutrition/the-paleo-diet.aspx

Paleo Diet. (2015). US News. https://health.usnews.com/best-diet/paleo-diet

Perry, A. (2017, January 24). *How to Choose Your Best Diet Plan (5 Factors to Consider)*. Anya Perry. https://anyaperry.com/nutrition/choose-best-diet-plan/

Petre, A. (2016a). *The Vegan Diet — A Complete Guide for Beginners*. Healthline. https://www.healthline.com/nutrition/vegan-diet-guide

Petre, A. (2016b, September 23). *6 Science-Based Health Benefits of Eating Vegan*. Healthline. https://www.healthline.com/nutrition/vegan-diet-benefits

Pfizer. (2017, September 4). *5 Things to Consider When Choosing a Diet*. Health24. https://www.health24.com/Lifestyle/Healthy-you/5-things-to-consider-when-choosing-a-diet-20170904

Pike, A. (2019, October 25). *What is the Flexitarian Diet?* International Food Information Council. https://foodinsight.org/what-is-the-flexitarian-diet/

Robertson, S. (2019, February 27). *Paleo Diet: Pros and Cons.* News Medical. https://www.news-medical.net/health/Paleo-Diet-Pros-and-Cons.aspx

Skyword. (2012). *How to Customize A Diet Plan to Meet Your Specific Needs*. STACK. https://www.stack.com/a/customize-diet-plan

Smith, A. (2020, April 27). *What to Know About Vegan Diets.* Medical News Today. https://www.medicalnewstoday.com/articles/149636

Smith, M., Robinson, L., & Segal, R. (2019). *The Mediterranean Diet*. Help Guide. https://www.helpguide.org/articles/diets/the-mediterranean-diet.htm

Streit, L. (2020, January 1). *The Flexitarian Diet: A Detailed Beginner's Guide*. Well+Good. https://www.wellandgood.com/what-is-flexitarian/

Taub-Dix, B. (2019, January 3). *What Is a Flexitarian Diet? What to Eat and How to Follow the Plan*. Everyday Health. https://www.everydayhealth.com/diet-nutrition/diet/flexitarian-diet-health-benefits-food-list-sample-menu-more/

Taylor, L. G. (2020, January 15). *12 Tips on How to Start a Flexitarian Diet and Stick To it*. Mums At The Table. https://www.mumsatthetable.com/start-flexitarian-diet

Topp, S. (2019, August 16). *5 Tips For Becoming Flexitarian*. Generation T. https://generationt.asia/self/5-tips-on-becoming-flexitarian

UPMC. (2016, April 2). *Pros and Cons of the Paleo Diet*. UPMC HealthBeat. https://share.upmc.com/2016/04/pros-cons-paleo-diet/

Valente, L. (2018, January 25). *9 Healthy Tips to Help You Start Eating a Vegan Diet*. Eating Well. http://www.eatingwell.com/article/279566/9-healthy-tips-to-help-you-start-eating-a-vegan-diet/

Watson, S. (2019, October 2). *What Is a Vegan Diet?* WebMD. https://www.webmd.com/diet/vegan-diet-overview#1

WebMD. (2019). *Slideshow: 12 Reasons to Love the Mediterranean Diet*. WebMD. https://www.webmd.com/diet/ss/slideshow-12-reasons-to-love-the-mediterranean-diet

Weeks, C. (2019, February 13). *20 Best Foods to Eat While Intermittent Fasting*. Eat This Not That. https://www.eatthis.com/intermittent-fasting-diet-foods/

Younkin, L. (2018, October 15). *Complete Keto Diet Food List: What You Can and Cannot Eat If You're on a Ketogenic Diet*. Eating Well. http://www.eatingwell.com/article/291245/complete-keto-diet-food-list-what-you-can-and-cannot-eat-if-youre-on-a-ketogenic-diet/

Younkin, L. (2019a). *Mediterranean Diet for Beginners: Everything You Need to Get Started*. Eating Well. http://www.eatingwell.com/article/291120/mediterranean-diet-for-beginners-everything-you-need-to-get-started/

Younkin, L. (2019b, April 11). *The Complete Paleo Diet Food List: What to Eat and What to Avoid*. Eating Well. http://www.eatingwell.com/article/290612/the-complete-paleo-diet-food-list-what-to-eat-and-what-to-avoid/

Zelman, K. M. (2007). *10 Tips for Finding the Best Diet That Works for You*. WebMD. https://www.webmd.com/diet/features/ten-tips-for-finding-the-best-diet-that-works-for-you#1